HEARING (OUR) VOICES:
PARTICIPATORY RESEARCH IN MENTAL HEALTH

Hearing (Our) Voices describes two innovative participatory action research projects – one on communication with medical professionals, the other on housing – carried out by a group of people diagnosed with schizophrenia. Under the guidance of Professor Barbara Schneider, participants designed the research, conducted interviews and focus groups, and participated in data analysis. Collectively, the participants disseminated the findings of the study through a number of creative strategies involving various media, including theatre performances, a documentary film, a graphic novel, and a travelling exhibit.

One of the central and significant findings of these projects is that people diagnosed with schizophrenia are frequently caught in a struggle between their dependence on care and their desire to lead independent lives. *Hearing (Our) Voices* points to ways to resolve this dilemma and thus transform lives by actively including people diagnosed with schizophrenia in research, in decision-making about their own treatment and housing, and in public discourse about schizophrenia.

BARBARA SCHNEIDER is an associate professor in the Communication Studies Program at the University of Calgary.

BARBARA SCHNEIDER

Hearing (Our) Voices

Participatory Research in Mental Health

UNIVERSITY OF TORONTO PRESS
Toronto Buffalo London

ISBN 978-1-4426-4071-9 (cloth)
ISBN 978-1-4426-1010-1 (paper)

∞

Printed on acid-free, 100% post-consumer recycled paper with
vegetable-based inks.

Library and Archives Canada Cataloguing in Publication

Schneider, Barbara, 1948–
Hearing (our) voices : participatory research in mental health /
Barbara Schneider.

Includes bibliographical references and index.
ISBN 978-1-4426-4071-9 (bound).   ISBN 978-1-4426-1010-1 (pbk.)

1. Schizophrenics – Services for – Alberta – Calgary – Case studies.
2. People with mental disabilities – Means of communication –
Alberta – Calgary – Case studies.   3. Schizophrenics – Housing –
Alberta – Calgary – Case studies.   4. Participant observation –
Case studies.   I. Title.

HV3008.C3S36 2009   362.2'04209712338   C2009-906276-3

This book has been published with the help of a grant from the Canadian
Federation for the Humanities and Social Sciences, through the Aid to
Scholarly Publications Program, using funds provided by the Social
Sciences and Humanities Research Council of Canada.

University of Toronto Press acknowledges the financial assistance to its
publishing program of the Canada Council for the Arts and the Ontario
Arts Council.

 Canada Council   Conseil des Arts
for the Arts   du Canada

 ONTARIO ARTS COUNCIL
CONSEIL DES ARTS DE L'ONTARIO

University of Toronto Press acknowledges the financial support for its
publishing activities of the Government of Canada through the Book
Publishing Industry Development Program (BPIDP).

Contents

Acknowledgments

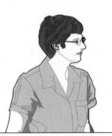

First and foremost, I thank the members of the Unsung Heroes who took part in the research projects described in this book. Without them there would have been nothing to write about. The research was a success because of their dedication and commitment to the work we undertook together. Also involved in the projects were several research assistants from the Graduate Program in Communications Studies at the University of Calgary: Hannah Scissons, Monique Solomon, and Concetta Ranieri took part in the project at various times and contributed to the writing of this book. Michelle Coyne coded the data in the housing project. I thank them for helping me to think about what we were doing together. Graduate students Tom Everrett and Everett Wilson contributed their brilliant artistic talents in making the DVD and creating the project website. Technical designer Colin McDonald created the photovoice poster and the graphics and layout for the illustrated poster book and travelling exhibit. Without the help of these gifted and dedicated artists, we could not have produced all the wonderful materials we did. Thanks to the Schizophrenia Society of Alberta, Calgary Chapter, for providing a meeting room and lots of encouragement. Thanks also to my friends and colleagues who read drafts of the book and provided invaluable feedback: Eileen Coughlan, Robert Seiler, Liza McCoy, and Jo-Anne Andre, and to my mother, Miriam Schneider, who worked her way through a complete draft. And finally, I thank the Killam Trust at the University of Calgary for granting me a fellowship that gave me the luxury of freedom from teaching and other duties so I could complete the writing of this book.

HEARING (OUR) VOICES:
PARTICIPATORY RESEARCH IN MENTAL HEALTH

Prologue

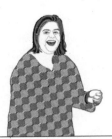

In this book, I tell the story of two participatory action research projects carried out by a group of people diagnosed with schizophrenia. Participatory action research involves members of a community group in conducting research on a topic of interest and relevance to them. People directly impacted by the problem being studied become co-researchers involved in every aspect of the investigation, from initiating the project, choosing the topic, and designing the research, to gathering and analysing the data and disseminating and using the results. Our projects were carried out over eight years by a group of people who chose two research topics that were of critical importance to them: communication between people diagnosed with schizophrenia and their medical professionals; and housing for people diagnosed with schizophrenia. They designed the research, conducted interviews and focus groups with others who have been diagnosed with schizophrenia, participated in data analysis, and took an active role in disseminating the research results.

This book has a number of interrelated goals. Perhaps first and foremost is to describe a successful example of participatory action research that involves people with a diagnosis of schizophrenia. A general presumption exists that people diagnosed with schizophrenia are unreliable, cognitively challenged, lacking in judgment, and unable to be full participants in society. Our projects demonstrate the falsity of this presumption and show that, in spite of the considerable challenges faced by people diagnosed with schizophrenia, they can make a significant contribution to understanding medical and housing issues for people with mental health diagnoses. As one of the people who took part says whenever he is asked about his contribution to the projects,

'I know that this research will refute the notion that people diagnosed with schizophrenia are unproductive members of society.' He speaks not just from his knowledge of negative understandings of schizophrenia prevalent among the general public but from his own experience of being told repeatedly by his service providers that he would never amount to anything in his life. He is now a published writer with a regular column in *Schizophrenia Digest*, a national Canadian magazine, and articles in various publications including the *Calgary Herald*, the primary newspaper in Calgary.[1]

A second goal is to contribute to the literature on communication between people diagnosed with schizophrenia and their medical service providers and to the literature on housing for people with mental health diagnoses. Participatory action research stands in sharp contrast to traditional research on schizophrenia, which has generally been carried out by people who have a professional or academic interest in mental health issues. People diagnosed with schizophrenia are the objects of study in this kind of research; they provide the raw material, whether biological, psychological, social, or cultural, for interpretation by those doing the research. While research carried out by professionals and academics has produced a tremendous amount of valuable knowledge about schizophrenia, it has also excluded people diagnosed with schizophrenia themselves as legitimate contributors to the production of this knowledge. Even in qualitative research, the goal of which is to understand schizophrenia from the perspective of those who experience it, people diagnosed with schizophrenia have typically had very little to say about which topics are researched, what questions are asked, how the research is carried out, and how the results are disseminated and used. A participatory approach in which people directly impacted by the problem being studied are involved in every aspect of the research has the potential to produce knowledge about the perspectives and experiences of people themselves that is not available in any other way.

An additional goal is to make a case for and illustrate our use of non-traditional research dissemination strategies. Academic research is generally published in peer-reviewed academic journals and books, which are often inaccessible to non-academic audiences. We did not want our work to disappear into the journals never to be seen by anyone unfamiliar with these publications. We have therefore used a number of dissemination strategies to reach a wide variety of audiences. These include readers' theatre performances, a documentary film, a photo poster, an illustrated poster book, a travelling exhibit based on the poster book, and a website. We hope that this description of our research and dissemination activities will help academics and practitioners who want to do something similar to succeed in their research projects. We also hope that people with a diagnosis of schizophrenia themselves, their families and friends and perhaps even a more general audience will be interested in what we have done.

Who We Are

Before beginning, I want to introduce the characters who appear in the story. These include thirteen members of a support group for people diagnosed with schizophrenia called the Unsung Heroes Peer Support Group, run by the Schizophrenia Society of Alberta, Calgary Chapter. They carried out the research projects with my guidance and support. The members of the Unsung Heroes know better than anyone what it is like to live with schizophrenia. They are all currently diagnosed with schizophrenia or schizoaffective disorder,[2] although many have received various diagnoses over the years, a source of considerable frustration to them. Among them, they have many years of experience of being on the receiving end of treatment and services from people and organizations trying to help them: the mental health and housing systems, their family members, psychiatrists, psychologists, social workers, psychiatric nurses, emergency room personnel, and countless others. Four people took part in both projects: Michele Misurelli, Laurie Arney, George Benson, and Mark Sunderland; three took part only in the first: Dana Nickerson, Ken Lucas, and one person who chose not to be included in this book; five took part only in the second: Mary Mitchell, Jamal Ali, Cindy Calderbank, Claude Mathieu, and Dale Silbernagel; Suzan Desserud joined us to work on the illustrated poster book. Each person brought something to the projects. Some were good at interviewing, some were good at being interviewed, some were good at offering ideas in the discussions, some were good at performing in our readers' theatre presentations. As with any group, each person made a unique contribution without any one of which the projects would have been diminished.

Jamal Ali became part of the research group because he wanted to know what participatory action research was like. He enjoys building relationships with colleagues in the group and is described by others as outspoken, eager, and an eloquent speaker. He hopes this research project will help convince those in positions of authority to build more affordable housing for people with mental illnesses. Jamal's writing has been published in the *Schizophrenia Digest, Calgary Herald, Alexandra Musings*, and numerous local and provincial newsletters. Friends and family are very important to Jamal. His other interests include table tennis and arts and crafts.

Laurie Arney is an artist and mother of two grown daughters. She teaches arts and crafts at the Schizophrenia Society, where she is also a peer support outreach worker. Her other interests are writing, walking, and crochet, which she teaches to others. She loves to paint fairies and flowers. Laurie maintains her wellness by trying to reduce stress in her life and by doing things that are meaningful to her. As an artist, Laurie brings creativity and compassionate insight to the research project. Known for her gift for saying the right thing at the right time, Laurie enjoys the chance to talk about subjects that don't normally get talked about and feels she is helping to make a difference. Through being part of the research group, she has learned that she is not alone. This experience has confirmed for her how important it is to feel heard. She hopes the research will make changes to the way homeless people are treated.

George Benson keeps a busy social schedule in addition to being part of the research group. He enjoys meeting with friends over coffee. Members of the research group appreciate George's questioning, caring, and reliable approach. For George, participating in the research projects meant that he learnt more communication skills. He hopes that this work will make him a 'more enlightened person, enlightening to others and a reflection of myself.' George attends the Calgary Association of Self Help and the Canadian Mental Health Association's drop-in activities. He also attends Foothills Hospital sports activities. He enjoys swimming, walking, and making model cars.

Cindy Calderbank feels lucky to have had a chance to belong to the group and enjoy the camaraderie while making a difference for people struggling with mental illness and homelessness. She recently wrote an article for the *Schizophrenia Digest* about advocating for herself. Cindy attends programs at the Calgary Association of Self Help and learns about computers at Ability Society. She is interested in flying small aircraft and in survival techniques. She loves all kinds of music and believes you should never belittle yourself or others.

Suzan Desserud joined the Research Group after watching the 'Hearing (Our) Voices' DVD. Her experience in public speaking enabled her to join the presentations and answer questions about schizophrenia. She has been a member of the Schizophrenia Society in Calgary since 1985 and is active in several of their programs. Suzan has a Bachelor of Fine Arts and enjoys doing pencil drawings of scenery and animals. She also has been writing in her journals for years. Suzan is noted for her intelligence, creativity, and positive energy, which uplifts the group. She copes with having schizophrenia by managing the amount of stress in her life carefully.

Ken Lucas joined the research group to find out about participatory research. He enjoys doing the presentations and especially going on the out-of-town trips. The friendships of group members mean a lot to him. Others find Ken caring, outgoing, and supportive. Ken attends Potential Place Clubhouse and the Unsung Heroes Peer Support Group. Ken's other activities are swimming and bowling with friends. He likes football and hockey. Ken also likes to help others who are coping with schizophrenia and says that helping others helps him to keep well.

Claude Mathieu's goals for the research are to 'bring awareness to those in need as well as to potential providers and benefactors.' He also wants to make a contribution towards helping others to cope with their illness and symptoms. A man of strong values and principles, he is described by others in the group as compassionate, considerate, and analytical. His participation in the group has encouraged him to be at ease in many aspects of his life. Claude is past president of the Unsung Heroes Peer Support Program and does volunteer work for his church and the Schizophrenia Society. He enjoys playing bridge.

Michele Misurelli is employed by the Schizophrenia Society as the coordinator of the Unsung Heroes program. She also took on the job of being the main contact for the members of the research group. Michele brought a warm balance of passion, empathy, caring, and dependability to the projects. She is passionate about her desire to improve the quality of life for people suffering from schizophrenia and generous with her time when it comes to helping members of the Unsung Heroes group or others in the community. Michele would like to see more bricks and mortar in the form of 3500 more subsidized apartments in Calgary to house the homeless and 5000 more subsidized single-dwelling homes. Aside from her involvement with the Unsung Heroes and the research projects, Michele is raising a sixteen-year-old daughter, Jennifer.

Mary Mitchell values the strengths of the research group and feels that as a group we can have more power to change the housing situation. Mary's goal for the research is that it will help to find ways to create more stable housing for people diagnosed with schizophrenia. She hopes this research will provide meaningful ideas that others can draw on. Mary has recently become the first woman president of the Unsung Heroes Peer Support Group. Her confidence and positive attitude have brought a steadiness and reliability to the Unsung Heroes support group for a number of years. In the future Mary would like to be involved in another project that would reduce the stigma around mental illness.

Dana Nickerson took part in the first research project mainly to enlighten medical professionals about the patients' point of view and to open them up to new ideas. She is known for the volunteer work she does for the Schizophrenia Society and Potential Place Clubhouse. She is a peer support outreach worker whose wisdom and ability as a good listener allow her to be a mentor to others with schizophrenia, helping them to help themselves. Dana is an artist and enjoys drawing wildlife. She also makes jewellery and has started painting and drawing portraits. Dana loves all life, especially animals. She recently adopted two cats.

Dale Silbernagel is the strong, silent, thoughtful member of the research group. He doesn't say much, but when he does, he makes a significant contribution. Dale learned to operate our video camera and became the group's official videographer, taping many of the meetings and interviews. Dale became part of the research group because he wanted to learn something new. Through his participation in the research, Dale came to understand that people who are homeless do not choose this way of life, but end up without a home often through circumstances that are beyond their control. He hopes that the research will help to change how people who are homeless are perceived in society. Dale volunteers many hours of his time at the Schizophrenia Society helping with their computer systems. He is also a peer mentor for the peer options program at the Canadian Mental Health Association. Dale likes working with metal and tools.

Mark Sunderland took part in the research to help to educate people about the difficult things that are part of the experience of mental illness. He hopes the project will help to 'stop the inhumanity in the mental health system.' The other members in the group appreciate Mark as a serious, kind, friendly, and courageous person. For him, coping with schizophrenia is a full-time job. To help himself keep well, he exercises and stays away from too much junk food. He enjoys visiting with friends, eating out, and going to movies. He has a special interest in architecture and music and enjoys window-shopping and visiting art galleries. Mark likes where he lives right now and he strives to be as happy as possible.

Barbara Schneider: I am an associate professor in the Department of Communication and Culture at the University of Calgary where I conduct research and teach in the Communications Studies program. Although I have considerable experience in various kinds of research, I claim no professional expertise in schizophrenia. My academic training is in biology, music, communications studies, and education. My connection to schizophrenia is as the mother of a son who was diagnosed with schizophrenia in 2000, when he was twenty-three. This happened about two weeks before I was offered my job as a professor at the University of Calgary. When the dean called late on a Friday afternoon to tell me that I was the selection committee's choice, I stood in stunned silence holding the phone, thinking, 'I can't do both. I can't be both the mother of a person diagnosed with schizophrenia and a university researcher and teacher.' I didn't say this to her. Instead, I recovered and graciously (I hope) accepted the job. In the years since, I have continued to feel tension between my two worlds. In one I am a concerned mother, coping with a challenging illness in my family, dealing with the loss of my dreams and hopes for my son, and taking up my role as a lifelong support for him. In the other, I am a communications scholar with a particular interest in listening to stories and understanding the experiences of people in various situations. I saw an opportunity to bring my two worlds together when, in early 2001, I came across a call for grant proposals from the Canadian Centre on Disability Studies for participatory action research involving people with disabilities. I had already begun doing research on the social and cultural aspects of schizophrenia, and this seemed a natural way to extend what I was doing. Before the projects described in this book, I had been a solo researcher, conceiving and carrying out both traditional and non-traditional projects on my own.[3] My role in the projects described here was to provide a framework for the members of the Unsung Heroes to take part and to make their contributions. I became the facilitator of their research ideas, making it possible for them to become co-researchers in the fullest sense of the word.

All of the Unsung Heroes members are very committed to participating in any research that might have the potential to make sense of schizophrenia and help others like themselves to suffer less. When I first approached them, they had some idea of what participating in traditional kinds of research might involve – many had given blood and fingerprints to University of Calgary researchers investigating bio-chemical aspects of schizophrenia; others had filled out surveys about their current and preferred living situations for a small study on hous-ing for people with mental health diagnoses in Calgary. They had no idea of what a participatory action research project might ask of them. In fact, I confess that I too had no real idea of what the projects would ask of either them or me. And none of us had any idea at all of what our work together would give us in return. Our decision to pursue a grant and to begin working together sent us off on an eight-year research journey that has taken us to places we never imagined.

1 Introduction

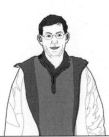

'This research is a breakthrough for us. It's a unique experience for us, and it's a model for the world.' —Jamal Ali

Before beginning the story of our research projects, I want to introduce some of the ideas that underlie our work. I begin with an overview of our projects and follow this with a discussion of participatory action research and an introduction to narrative. I then present a description of schizophrenia and a brief review of literature on communication with medical professionals and on housing for people with psychiatric diagnoses. The plot of our story – what we did, how we did it, what we learned, how we told others about what we learned, and how our lives were changed – will unfold in the succeeding chapters. I hope, by the end, that you will be convinced of the worth of the whole enterprise. Our work is a call for the inclusion of people diagnosed with schizophrenia in research, in decision-making about medical treatment, housing, and other aspects of their lives, and in public discourse about schizophrenia. It is a call to change public perceptions of people diagnosed with schizophrenia and to improve their treatment in the mental health and housing systems.

History of the Projects

Over a period of eight years, the members of the Unsung Heroes and I undertook two research projects together. The first was on communication between people diagnosed with schizophrenia and their medical professionals; the second was on housing for people diagnosed with schizophrenia.

Communication between People Diagnosed with Schizophrenia and Their Medical Professionals

The first project was prompted by the call for grant proposals from the Canadian Centre on Disability Studies. I contacted the woman then serving as executive director of the Schizophrenia Society in Calgary to ask if the society would be interested in collaborating on a participatory research project. She was very enthusiastic and put me in touch with the Unsung Heroes Peer Support Group. I attended two meetings of the group to discuss with members whether some of them would be interested in working on a project that would involve them as co-researchers and, if so, what they might be interested in doing. Together we wrote a proposal for a project that would investigate some aspect of how people cope with having schizophrenia. We were successful in getting a small grant.

This project took us two years. As we describe in more detail in the next chapter, the seven people who took part as co-researchers conducted in-depth interviews with each other and with a few additional people from the Unsung Heroes about their experiences in the mental health system. We produced a readers' theatre presentation based on the research data that the group members performed for various groups of mental health professionals in Calgary and the surrounding area. We also co-wrote an article about the project that was published in an academic journal.[1]

Housing for People Diagnosed with Schizophrenia

Over the course of the first project, group members went from thinking of themselves as people upon whom others carry out various kinds of research to thinking of themselves as people who can themselves carry out research and in so doing make a significant contribution to society. As the first project was winding down, group members expressed an interest in doing another project, this time on housing for people diagnosed with schizophrenia. They regarded this as a significant problem, both from their personal experiences and from their observations of others' experiences. I saw an opportunity to apply to the Homelessness and Diversity in Canada Program of the Social Sciences and Humanities Research Council of Canada (SSHRC) for funds to carry out this project. We again wrote a proposal and when we received this grant began work on the second project. This project, much more ambitious than the first, took us five years.

With our experience in the first project under our belts and with the generous funding from SSHRC, our accomplishments in the second project exceeded anything we might have imagined when we started. This time nine people were involved. We not only conducted interviews within the research group, we also talked to many people outside the group both in individual interviews and in focus groups. We carried out a photovoice project in which some members of the research group took photos of their homes and communities to illustrate what home means to them. The poster resulting from the photo project was given to numerous agencies in Calgary. We again produced a readers' theatre presentation, which group members continue to perform. We made a thirty-minute documentary film about the project, which has been seen in communities and classrooms around the world. With an additional grant from SSHRC, we produced an illustrated poster book based on the research findings from both projects. We received yet another grant, this time from Human Resources and Social Development Canada (HRSDC), to turn our poster book into a travelling exhibit that has been shown in cities across Canada. All of these activities are described on a website that makes our materials widely available (http://callhome.ucalgary.ca).

Participatory Action Research

Participatory action research has been described as 'a democratic process concerned with developing practical knowing in the pursuit of worthwhile human purposes.'[2] It is embedded in a tradition of cooperative inquiry that emphasizes working with community groups as co-researchers.[3] This approach is quite different from the traditional scientific approach to knowledge generation, which places the academic researcher at a distance from the subjects of the research in order to produce 'objective' knowledge. The participatory approach assumes that the experts are the people who live the experiences that are being studied. And it assumes that knowledge is produced through the active engagement and interaction of all participants in the research. Participatory research strives to transform the social relations of research[4] by regarding participants as both co-researchers and co-subjects. It is often described as having an emancipatory or empowerment agenda, particularly as a way to improve the lives of the people involved and others like them.[5] Three interrelated goals of participatory action research include the production of practical knowledge that will be useful to people in their everyday lives; action to use this knowledge to have a positive effect on the lives of others; and, ideally, transformation in the lives of the people who take part.

As participatory action research is a philosophy of engagement in the research process rather than a research method, it does not direct researchers to particular research sites or methods. Its proponents work in a range of organizational and community settings and use both quantitative and qualitative research strategies. They conduct traditional surveys and interviews and they also use innovative research strategies such as community mapping.[6] We join a small but growing number of groups doing what is variously called mental health consumer- or service user-led research, research that involves people with experience in the mental health system in meaningful ways.[7] Examples of such research projects can be found in the so-called grey literature, on websites and in organizational reports, and in academic journals. Following is a partial list of such studies.[8]

- The California Network of Mental Health Clients, a group of people with experience in the mental health system, developed and administered a study involving interviews, focus groups, and a state-wide survey of people who use mental health services to investigate what promotes or harms the well-being of people with mental health problems. [9]
- The Bridge to Discharge Project, a participatory research project in Canada, resulted in a program designed to help people diagnosed with schizophrenia integrate successfully back into the community after long-term hospitalization.[10]
- A group of researchers at Yale University used a participatory approach to involve people diagnosed with schizophrenia in exploring reasons for relapse and designing a program to help people avoid it.[11]
- Consumer Quality Initiatives (CQI), a service user-led research organization in Massachusetts, involves people who have experience with the mental health system in leading, designing, and carrying out survey research aimed at giving mental health service users a greater voice and larger role in their treatment.[12]

- Research that involves mental health service users in the United Kingdom has evaluated services from the users' perspective,[13] investigated people's own strategies for living with mental health problems,[14] and examined hospital psychiatric care.[15]
- Two recent books, *The Handbook of Service User Involvement in Mental Health Research*[16] and *This Is Survivor Research*,[17] describe various aspects of service user involvement in research and provide examples of and practical advice on carrying out such research.

This work has done much to establish the legitimacy and usefulness of research carried out by people who have experienced the mental health system. These studies have demonstrated that research in which people have control over the research questions that will be asked and how they will be answered produces credible and useful knowledge. In addition, such research gives people a mechanism for increasing self-determination and returning to a productive role in society. It enables people diagnosed with schizophrenia to become more aware of their own strengths and abilities, to see themselves in a new light, and therefore to reclaim a sense of themselves as worthwhile individuals. As participatory research is fundamentally about 'the right to speak,'[18] it offers people diagnosed with schizophrenia a way to both reclaim a positive identity and make a contribution to society.

Narrative

We have chosen a narrative approach in our projects, as our central focus was on the experiences and stories of the people who took part. In the interviews and focus groups we conducted, we collected the narratives of people who agreed to share their private stories with us. We then took these private stories and transformed them into a public story through the various modes of dissemination that we describe in chapter 6. And now in this book, I present the narrative of our research experiences. But narrative is much more than simply the telling of stories. It is also a way of knowing and a way of creating community. In fact, rhetorician Walter Fisher believes that all forms of human communication are narrative at heart and that knowledge is 'ultimately configured narratively.'[19] 'Knowledge,' he says, 'is found in the stories we tell one another.'[20] He believes that 'we experience and comprehend life as a series of ongoing narratives,'[21] and that all forms of communication may be seen as narrative in this broader sense. By this, he does not mean that all communication takes the form of the genre we call narrative; rather, he believes that narrative provides 'a conceptual frame that would account for the "stories" we tell each other – whether such "stories" are in the form of argumentation, narration, exposition, or aesthetic writing and performance.'[22] And no form of discourse (for example, science or logic) can be elevated above others 'because its form is predominantly argumentative.'[23] I call here on narrative, both in its more limited definition as the telling of stories and in its broader definition as the means through which we perceive the world and communicate with others, to provide a framework for our research activities and our stories about those activities.

Fisher's assertion that narrative is the basis of community is also important for our story. 'Communities,' he says, 'are co-constituted through communicative transactions in which participants co-author a story' that has meaning for them.[24] Fisher describes 'genuine communication as an ideal transaction, one of uncoerced, mutual, educative exchange'[25] and quotes Dewey, saying that communication is 'a process of sharing experience till it becomes a common possession. It modifies the disposition of both parties who partake in it.'[26] This understanding of communication is an ideal, perhaps impossible to truly achieve in any sphere of life, but it presents an ideal to strive for. It offers the possibility of relationships in which participants together negotiate meaning and construct a common story rather than simply accept the meanings and stories of those who appear to be higher in the traditional knowledge hierarchy.

Narrative also offers a way of asserting alternative versions of reality. Medical and popular versions of schizophrenia typically assign people diagnosed with schizophrenia negative identities that determine the kinds of stories about them that are expected and attended to. The stories of people diagnosed with schizophrenia themselves are typically ignored or discounted (theirs are 'crazy' stories), and their access to a public voice and audience is limited. Because narratives offer access to personal experiences, they encourage audiences to revise their perceptions of the narrators' experiences. By offering participants a public arena in which to tell their stories, projects such as ours give participants a way to change the public story that is told about them, to escape from the negative perceptions that others' stories attach to them, and to change how people diagnosed with schizophrenia are regarded and treated. We ask readers to hear the stories of the people who took part in these projects and to help us change the public story about schizophrenia.

Schizophrenia

Whenever we present our research, people ask, either in the question period or afterwards in private, for information about current thinking about schizophrenia. I think this hunger for information is indicative of the tremendous confusion that accompanies a diagnosis of schizophrenia both for those who receive the diagnosis and for their family members. Many people know that schizophrenia is widely considered to be the most severe and disabling mental illness.[27] Much less well known is the fact that many people diagnosed with schizophrenia can and do return to productive participation in society.

Schizophrenia is now firmly established as an illness, although this was not always the case. The very strangeness of the behaviours associated with madness has meant that there have been many ways of talking about schizophrenia over the centuries.[28] Now, in the early part of the twenty-first century, the medical version of schizophrenia as a brain illness, 'a broken brain,'[29] has become the dominant, perhaps the only available, discourse for understanding schizophrenia. However, a significant academic literature[30] and a consumer/psychiatric survivor activist social movement[31] both dispute the existence of schizophrenia as an identifiable medical entity, that is, as an illness. Adherents of this perspective point out that the causes of schizophrenia have not been identified, no medical test exists that can confirm its diagnosis, and no one set of symptoms is present in every case. They advocate the abandonment of all psychiatric diagnostic labels in describing the experiences and behaviours of people who come to be identified as having a mental illness and they promote the use of terms they regard as less stigmatizing, such as *mental health problems* or *mental distress* instead of mental illness.[32] Although I am sympathetic to these arguments, I continue to use the word *schizophrenia* as this is the word, along with the term *mental illness*, used by the co-researchers in these projects and the people they interviewed. But I want to acknowledge this ontological debate and do so by describing the people involved in this research as people diagnosed with schizophrenia – that is, as people whose experiences and behaviours have led to their involvement in the mental health system and to a consequent diagnosis of schizophrenia.

I also use the term mental health *service user* rather than consumer, as that is the term that predominates in the literature on the involvement of health services recipients in research and treatment decision-making, although it too is problematic as it defines people in terms of their use of mental health services, something they may not see as their primary identity. While I acknowledge the difficulties of using the word *schizophrenia*, our research is an attempt to change the meanings of this word by demonstrating the ability of people diagnosed with schizophrenia to make a significant contribution to knowledge about schizophrenia. The following description of schizophrenia is offered not to buttress the position that schizophrenia is a real medical entity, but to provide a context widely accepted in the mental health field within which the experiences of the people involved in our projects unfold.

It is widely agreed that schizophrenia can be identified in slightly less than 1 per cent of the population worldwide. This is approximately 300,000 people in Canada and 2.2 million people in the US. Although schizophrenia has been around for a long time,[33] it is still mysterious, surrounded by fear and misconception. One of the most common misconceptions about schizophrenia is that it involves split or multiple personalities. Schizophrenia is unrelated to split or multiple personalities. The combination of the Greek words *schizo* (split) and *phrene* (mind) was intended to refer to the fragmentation of mental processes, not to the splitting of the mind or personality itself.[34] Another misconception is the idea that, if people would just pull themselves together and exercise a little self-control, they could behave normally. As with all mental health problems, it is, of course, not at all so simple.

Hallucinations and delusions are probably the best-known experiences associated with schizophrenia. However, it also involves neurocognitive problems that can persist even when the psychotic experiences are reduced or controlled by medications. [35] These problems can make it hard for people to concentrate, think clearly, make decisions, solve problems, and remember things. People may also be unable to maintain personal hygiene or express normal emotions and may have reduced interest and motivation to take part in activities of daily life. Auditory hallucinations, in which people hear voices when there is no apparent source of the sound, are one of the hallmark experiences of schizophrenia. Voices may be friendly, but more commonly they are hostile and may direct the person to do something specific, such as jump off a building. People can also experience hallucinations in other sensory modes – sight, touch, taste, and smell. They can also experience delusions, or fixed and sometimes strange beliefs that are maintained in spite of evidence to the contrary, in which they typically believe that someone is controlling their life or that their brain is being directed by aliens or hostile governments.

This brief description does very little to convey the impact schizophrenia can have on a person's life. Certainly the personal and social effects of schizophrenia can be as troubling as the experiences of the illness itself. It 'causes people to feel disconnected from themselves, from others, from their environments, and from meaning and purpose in life.'[36] Many people isolate themselves from others as a result. They may be unable to maintain employment or housing, make or keep friends, or maintain long-term love relationships. The social stigma of a diagnosis of schizophrenia may also contribute to their isolation from society. The powerful medications taken by people diagnosed with schizophrenia can have debilitating side effects, including weight gain, lethargy, vision problems, elevated blood sugar, increased risk of diabetes, constipation, dizziness, loss of sexual drive, headaches, hair loss, and involuntary movements. Schizophrenia is, in short, much more than the sum of its symptoms.

In the past, a diagnosis of schizophrenia was often seen as the end of hope for normal participation in society. Schizophrenia was thought to have a downhill course with no chance of remission,[37] and people were often told by their medical practitioners to give up any thoughts of returning to their previous lives and activities.[38] The legacy of this perspective is a mental health system that typically treats people in a highly controlling and paternalistic way, removing from them basic human rights for choice and self-determination in their own treatment and lives. Although this is slowly starting to change,[39] psychiatrists and other mental health professionals typically regard people diagnosed with schizophrenia as severely impaired and unable to make decisions for themselves. They believe they know what is best for people and expect to be in control of treatment. People diagnosed with schizophrenia are expected to be acquiescent recipients of treatments and services designed to help them cope with having schizophrenia, and others, particularly mental health professionals, but also family members and friends, feel entitled to speak about and for them. In the face of this paternalistic and dismissive perspective, people diagnosed with schizophrenia have had an uphill battle in establishing meaningful lives – in living 'outside'[40] the totalizing identity imposed by a diagnosis of schizophrenia.

Evidence that the traditional view held by the mental health system is not the only possible story for people diagnosed with schizophrenia comes from two threads of literature that developed in the 1980s. One thread was first-person accounts by people who described their experiences of being diagnosed and treated in the mental health system and their emergence from these experiences to productive lives. Pat Deegan's story is an example.[41] She was diagnosed with schizophrenia at age seventeen. After many years of despair, during which she sat in a chair and smoked, she found a way to resist the hopelessness and alienation produced by the diagnosis of schizophrenia and began to rebuild her life. She went on to get a PhD and become an advocate for better treatment for people identified as having mental illness. Accounts of this kind demonstrated that having a diagnosis of schizophrenia was not the end of productive participation in society. The other thread was the demonstration in a number of North American and international studies[42] that a diagnosis of schizophrenia was not a predictor of inevitable deterioration to permanent disability, as was commonly thought. Instead, these worldwide studies found tremendous heterogeneity among people diagnosed with schizophrenia. Some do indeed experience and struggle with cognitive and other impairments all their lives, but a substantial proportion are able to return to normal participation in activities of daily living and some recover completely and have no further need for medication or other treatments.

These two threads of literature form the background to what has come to be called the recovery movement.[43] Unlike the use of the term in the medical model, which typically understands recovery to mean an end to or at least a reduction of symptoms and a return to a previous level of functioning, recovery in this usage is not necessarily synonymous with cure. Instead it is believed that people can have fulfilling lives although they may continue to experience symptoms and impairments of various kinds. The recovery movement seeks to return control and self-determination to those diagnosed with schizophrenia, encouraging them to be responsible for managing their own 'transformation from a mental patient or a disabled person to a person in recovery.'[44] The recovery movement does not exclude medical treatment or rehabilitation but rather encourages individuals to become active participants in rather than passive recipients of treatments and to use treatments and services to help them manage their symptoms and their lives. The words *hope, healing, empowerment,* and *connection* convey the central tenets of the recovery movement.[45]

Our projects offer further evidence that people diagnosed with schiz-ophrenia, including those experiencing ongoing challenges, are not just 'bundles of pathologies,' but are people first, with abilities, strengths, and potential for growth, just like people who have not been diagnosed with schizophrenia. They are well able to offer significant insights into their own situations and experiences, to identify the kinds of treatment and support that will enable them to rebuild their lives, to contribute to the production of knowledge about schizophrenia, and to advocate for change in how people diagnosed with schizophrenia are treated. The participatory action research approach that we took in our projects offered an ideal way to harness their experience and expertise and to engage them in generating knowledge that can contribute to improving the situations of others like themselves.

Communication between People Diagnosed with Schizophrenia and Their Medical Professionals

The centrality of communication in relationships between health care providers and people diagnosed with schizophrenia may seem some-what obvious. Indeed, the amount of research and practitioner inter-est in the burgeoning field of doctor/patient communication signals that many people are concerned about and want to improve this form of communication.[46] However, many doctors and other mental health professionals do not conceptualize their relationships with their pa-tients in terms of the quality of their interactions with them. This be-came clear to us in the presentation phase of our first project. At one presentation, an older psychiatrist rose to express his dismay that the younger doctors in his program had not attended our presentation. In his view, many of them did not understand the importance of commu-nication and had never really listened to their patients long enough to hear and respond to their points of view on their own lives and treat-ments.

We are certainly not the first to suggest that a good relationship with health care practitioners is important for those who are diagnosed with schizophrenia. Medication, although often an essential part of treat-ment, is but one factor in helping people diagnosed with schizophrenia to become well and to rebuild their lives. 'Strong patient-physician col-laboration'[47] is integral to the recovery process in schizophrenia and influences the outcome of treatment. The willingness of health care professionals to answer patients' questions and to provide information about schizophrenia and medications has been shown to be crucial to developing and maintaining an effective therapeutic relationship[48] and in leading to patient satisfaction with treatment experiences.[49] Studies have also shown that the development of trust between doctor and patient and willingness on the part of the doctor to offer choice and negotiate power are important in the treatment of schizophrenia.[50] These studies suggest that establishing a good working relationship is the responsibility of doctors and other mental health care practitioners.[51] Despite this research, a significant number of doctors do not tell patients when they are first diagnosed that they have schizophrenia,[52] thereby creating a conspiracy of silence around the diagnosis. Doctors also may prescribe medications without understanding and acknowledging the degree of patients' distress about the often-severe side effects.[53] Such actions damage the therapeutic relationship, thereby contributing to the continuing distress rather than to the recovery of people diagnosed with schizophrenia.

Housing for People Diagnosed with Schizophrenia

Providing housing for people with psychiatric diagnoses is widely regarded as extremely challenging, and it is generally agreed that a significant proportion of the homeless population consists of people who have or could have a psychiatric diagnosis.[54] They are the least likely subgoup of the homeless population to gain access to housing programs, and the threat of return to homelessness is ever-present.

Mounting evidence exists that this housing instability can be addressed through a variety of housing alternatives in combination with a range of support services. [55] A debate has developed in the literature, however, about how best to achieve stable living situations for people with psychiatric diagnoses.[56] Some programs favour a linear residential continuum model in which people are moved step-by-step through a progression of services (sometimes called 'treatment first'). Others favour a supported housing model in which people are placed immediately from the streets into independent living situations (sometimes called 'housing first'). The linear model generally involves a continuum of services including outreach to those who are homeless, treatment for both psychiatric and addiction problems, transitional housing, and finally independent housing. Programs of this sort generally require that individuals comply with requirements for psychiatric and addiction treatment before becoming eligible for housing. Once in housing, failure to participate in ongoing treatment generally results in loss of housing.[57] Critics point out that this model leads to frequent change of housing and therefore continuing instability in people's lives. They also point out that skills learned for success in one type of housing may not be transferable to another type of housing. Perhaps most importantly, the linear model deprives people of choice and freedom in housing and treatment because housing is contingent on accepting treatment.[58]

A number of studies[59] have shown that placing people with psychiatric diagnoses and substance abuse problems directly into independent housing situations without requiring either psychiatric treatment or sobriety produced excellent results in helping them to maintain stable housing. Researchers compared an innovative program that placed people directly from the streets into supported independent living situations with a traditional linear residential treatment program that moved people step by step into supervised independent living. They found that the innovative program was significantly more successful in reducing both hospitalizations and homelessness and incurred fewer costs. They also found that people housed in independent living situations were more likely to experience a higher degree of community integration.[60] In sum, this group of studies found that people with mental health and substance abuse problems were able to obtain and maintain independent housing in spite of their psychiatric and addiction problems.

There are no easy answers to the complex needs of people with psychiatric diagnoses, and no one solution will work for all such people. People with psychiatric diagnoses are not a homogeneous group about which useful generalizations can be made.[61] Evidence suggests, however, that people with psychiatric diagnoses are more likely to remain in housing if they feel satisfied with it and perceive it to be a good match with their needs.[62] Surveys indicate that people with psychiatric diagnoses prefer housing that is their own, affordable, permanent, and integrated into the community, and that offers flexible supports as needed.[63]

Inclusion of People Diagnosed with Schizophrenia

Our projects build on and contribute to the literatures on both communication and housing with qualitative research that takes the standpoint of people with mental health diagnoses themselves. Our central finding, identified by the people who took part as co-researchers, is a paradox in their lives that runs as a thread through all the work we did together. People diagnosed with schizophrenia are caught between their dependence on care and their longing for independent lives. Professionals and family members who help and care for them have a desire to help them, but also have authority and power over them. A relationship intended to be positive, enabling, and empowering is at the same time controlling and disempowering. People diagnosed with schizophrenia want and need care and support from mental health professionals, family members, government agencies, and housing and other social service providers to maintain stability in their lives. But they also want freedom from the paternalistic control that accompanies care, with the ability to make their own choices about medical treatments and how they will live. Acting on the desire for independence from medical and social service providers can jeopardize access to care. Readers not familiar with the world of mental health and illness may think I am exaggerating. But I can report that I was myself told by my son's psychiatrist, at an early stage in our acquaintance with schizophrenia, that if my son tried the alternative treatments I was exploring, he would no longer treat my son.

But our research projects do not tell a sad and resentful story of people trapped forever in this dependence/independence paradox, unable to overcome the requirement to behave in ways that will be seen as 'compliant' (sometimes defined by people on the receiving end of services as 'doing what you are told even when you don't want to') in order to maintain access to services. Ours is a hopeful story, one that points to a way to resolve this paradox and transform the lives of people diagnosed with schizophrenia. Our research shows the value, indeed the necessity, of including people diagnosed with schizophrenia in three areas – in research, in decision-making about their treatment and housing, and in public discourse about schizophrenia – to promote real change in the way people diagnosed with schizophrenia are treated and housed and to enable them to move beyond the dependence/independence paradox. Communication is central to achieving all three forms of inclusion.

Inclusion of people diagnosed with schizophrenia in all aspects of knowledge production about schizophrenia, that is, in research, has the potential to produce knowledge that is not available in any other way. People diagnosed with schizophrenia themselves know best about their experiences and what helps them to cope with these experiences. They are able to steer the research to the issues and concerns that are most important to them. Focusing the research in this way has the potential to provide information that can dramatically improve the care that people diagnosed with schizophrenia receive. As I discuss in the next chapter, issues of power and control loom large in participatory research and it is only through open and collegial communication as described by Fisher that these can be resolved and inclusion achieved.

The conclusions and recommendations that come from our research make it clear that what people diagnosed with schizophrenia most want and need in their care is inclusion as equal partners in decision-making about all aspects of their lives, including medical treatment and housing. The tension between care and control in their relationships with service providers produces dilemmas that they find themselves having to manage in all their interactions with their service providers. Including them as equal partners in decision-making about their treatment has the potential to mitigate these dilemmas and to make life easier not only for them but also for the people who care for them. This too can happen only through open and collegial communication.

Communication is also central to the inclusion of people diagnosed with schizophrenia in public discourse about schizophrenia. Successful inclusion in public discourse requires the use of modes of communication that are not traditionally used to disseminate academic research. Through our various dissemination strategies, the co-researchers in our projects have presented their results to diverse audiences, including psychiatrists, psychiatry residents, medical students, other mental health practitioners, scholars in various fields, people with mental health diagnoses, family members, and the general public. Without non-traditional modes of dissemination, the people involved in the projects could not have the public voice necessary to advocate for inclusion both in knowledge production activities and in decision-making about their own lives.

We promote the inclusion of people diagnosed with schizophrenia not just because it is the 'right' thing to do, but because in the long run it benefits everyone – people diagnosed with schizophrenia themselves, their medical and housing service providers, and society generally. These research projects empowered one small group of very marginalized people diagnosed with schizophrenia to speak directly to psychiatrists, other mental health professionals, and the general public

about their treatment and housing experiences. Through speaking publicly, they contribute to changing how they and others like themselves
are treated and to changing how people diagnosed with schizophrenia
are perceived. As a wonderful by-product of being involved in the research, particularly in the dissemination activities, they also contribute
to changing the circumstances of their own lives. They move beyond
the dependence/independence paradox and take their place as full
members in society, with the ability and right to speak about issues that
concern them.

Conclusion

Although we all gained something from our involvement in the
projects, the work we did together was not therapy. It was research.
I am not trained and have no personal or professional interest in providing therapy. If group members needed support of some kind, other
group members, some of them much more understanding and skilled
than I could ever hope to be, provided it. However, this does not mean
that the experiences we had together were not in some way beneficial
for everyone involved. In fact, the benefits we experienced are as important as the knowledge we produced, although they are a welcome
by-product rather than a direct goal of the projects. The projects offered
the people involved an opportunity to overcome the isolation so char-
acteristic of schizophrenia by meeting with others in the same situation to investigate topics of importance to us all. We found a sense of
connection as we became a supportive community through doing the
research. Although there were some difficult times, particularly during
the interview stage of the projects when the people being interviewed
talked about tragic circumstances in their lives, the research group
members continued to come to meetings and to listen to difficult stories. The project became an important part of all our lives as the feeling
that we were doing something significant that might have real and positive consequences for people diagnosed with schizophrenia motivated
us to stick with it.

One of my contributions to the projects has been to write most of the
material we have published. As the academic in the group, I was the
only person trained to write academically about research and the only
one with the inclination and financial support to do so. But the fact that
I was doing the writing excluded my co-researchers from participation
in the final stage of the research process – the presentation of our work

in written form for an academic and practitioner audience. This was a dilemma to which there was no easy solution. We handled it by agreeing that I would bring whatever I was writing to them so they could see what I was doing and approve it or suggest changes. We have done the same with this book, with group members providing feedback on early drafts.

In writing this book, I have drawn on academic literature in a number of fields, material generated in the research, and discussions among the group members. I have also drawn on the work of graduate research assistants who wrote drafts of portions of three chapters. In several chapters, I have included journal entries written by group members during the course of the projects. These journal entries give a sense of how the co-researchers experienced the research process. The journals were small hardbound books that I bought for each person in the groups. In the first project, we made time to write in the journals towards the end of each meeting. Many people found this quite challenging and some simply gave up. But a few liked this part of the project and wrote from time to time. In the second project, our meetings became so full and the project so busy that the journals just slipped away from us. We wrote after our meetings for the first couple of months, but after that, we never again managed to make time to write. I wrote occasionally in my own journal, but this became a struggle for me too as the research gathered intensity. Laurie was one of the few who liked writing in her journal in the first project. She continued to bring it to meetings during the second project and to write in it on her own time. Excerpts from her journal make a significant contribution to many sections of the book.

I have striven to stay true to the sensibilities of my co-researchers while presenting our work in a way that will be interesting, accessible, and useful. In the end, though, I am the author of this text. Although our research approach differs in significant ways from traditional research, I nevertheless use the language of research and stay within the conventions of academic writing to tell our story. I have structured the book and shaped each chapter in a recognizable academic way, offering a background of academic literature to introduce many of the chapters. My role as both an observer/narrator of and a participant in the research process complicates my task. So I also offer occasional commentary on the research from the perspective of a participant. As I discuss in chapter 6, even if I were not a participant, I could never be a neutral, omniscient observer, presenting our story 'as it really happened.' I am the creator of this representation of our research and I offer my apologies to my co-researchers if I have in some way misrepresented their voices and experiences. As the principles of participatory research remind us, true participation belongs to those who take part, not those who write about them.

2 What We Did (Method)

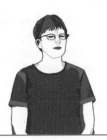

'After reading my transcript, I realized we accomplished two things. We were able to vent our feelings and we were able to speak about many issues that affected us. And hopefully we will make a difference in making changes to our system.' —Michele Misurelli

I begin our narrative with an account of what we did to carry out our research, from getting ethics approval for the projects and holding our first planning meetings to analysing our data.The description of the ways in which we disseminated our work appears in a later chapter. Here I describe how we accomplished the first level of inclusion, the involvement of people diagnosed with schizophrenia in the research. Before getting to the details of our projects, I explore the question of whether involvement of service users produces credible research. I also discuss a key methodological issue that relates to the interaction that takes place in the research process, namely power relations in this kind of research, including roles and levels of service user involvement.

Questions of Knowledge and Power

Some might wonder whether involving people with direct experience of the problem being studied produces 'good' research. Surely such an approach introduces 'bias' and reduces the 'objectivity' of the research. If a qualitative approach with a small sample size (like ours) is used, the research will not be representative of a diverse population of service users. In the age of 'evidence-based' policy and practice, the question arises whether service user involvement in research results in knowledge that is simply 'unscientific.'

The central question here is 'whose knowledge counts?' In traditional positivist approaches to research, which have dominated the field
of mental health, legitimate knowledge is produced by trained academic researchers using apparently neutral procedures to design and carry
out research. In this approach, researchers typically use measurement
and quantification to demonstrate the existence of causal relationships
that are presumed to operate independently of and often unbeknownst
to the individuals being studied. In order for knowledge to be reliable
and valid, it must be produced at a distance from those being studied,
with research subjects remaining in a passive role, so that any suspicion
of 'bias' that might 'contaminate' the results can be avoided.

Proponents of participatory research, on the other hand, believe all
researchers, including those who claim to be doing 'neutral' and 'objective' research, come to their work with attitudes, values, and perspectives that shape the questions they ask and the therefore the answers
they produce. Even participatory researchers who use traditional positivist methods themselves question the possibility of achieving objectivity and acknowledge the perspectives they bring to their research.
Those who advocate the use of qualitative methods also believe that
there is more to human life than can be captured through measurement.
They see the positivist tradition as just one way of making sense of
the social world. They believe that individual experience is an equally
important and valid source of knowledge, as people's lives are embedded in networks of personally meaningful relationships, not just
in causal relationships. Research that attends to individuals' own understandings of events and experiences and seeks to understand these
experiences from the individuals' own perspectives produces equally
important and credible knowledge. Rather than 'evidenced-based'
policy and practice, they use the term 'knowledge-based' policy and
practice,[1] and promote the involvement of individuals with experience
of the topic under study in producing practical knowledge that will be
useful to people in their everyday lives.

Proponents of participatory research believe not only that research in
this tradition is not 'bad' research, but that involving people with direct
experience of the problem being studied offers a way to improve the
quality and relevance of research.[2] It can ensure that research attends
to issues that are regarded as problematic by the people affected, not
just issues seen as problematic by researchers or service providers. It
likely increases the quality of the material collected, since people with
mental health issues may be more willing to reveal their experiences

(even in survey research) to people they see as having had similar experiences. A peer interviewer can put interviewees at ease and find a connection with them that a researcher without these experiences might not achieve. While this does not guarantee that interviewees will feel comfortable revealing difficult personal experiences, the fact that the interviewers are not people who might be in a position of authority over them (e.g., mental health care professionals doing research on the delivery of services) may enable them to say things they might not be able to say to authority figures. And involving people in data analysis ensures that results are interpreted in ways that remain true to the perspective of those being studied. If particular services have been studied, increasing the quality of the research by involving as co-researchers people with direct experience of those services can have a direct impact on the kind and quality of services offered and therefore have a positive impact on the lives of others.

Service user roles in research can be described on a continuum: advisory, consultation, collaboration, and control.[3] In the advisory role, service users are typically invited to be part of an advisory board in which their role is to represent the 'stakeholder group' of service users. They are usually outnumbered by health professionals and other interest groups and have minimal involvement in the design and conduct of the research. Consultation refers to situations in which service users are regarded as having knowledge or skills that are of value to the research project – they might be asked to help with designing a survey, for example – but control of all aspects of the research is retained by the professional researchers. Collaboration describes a situation in which service users collaborate with professional researchers on all aspects of the research, including topic selection, identification of the research question, design of the study, gathering and analysis of data, and dissemination of the findings. The final category, service user controlled research, is research that is initiated, directed, and led by service users. Professional researchers may be involved, but at the request of the service user researchers rather than as directors of the research.[4]

Our projects fall somewhere between collaboration and control. I initiated the first project, but the research group members initiated the second, and in both projects they had a significant degree of control over decision-making in all aspects of the research and dissemination. I became the facilitator, trainer, and supporter rather than the expert researcher, providing the information they needed to make decisions, but not making the decisions for them. Because I am not an expert in anything to do with mental health issues, I was in no position to be directive about the content of the research. However, there were times when I took an assertive role in the process of the research to keep the projects from bogging down. We negotiated ways to accomplish their goals without compromising the progress of the research. Looking back, I see my lack of professional training and expertise in mental health as a positive factor in the projects, enabling group members to grow into the role of content experts, as they later came to see themselves, without any 'competition' from me. I provided the research scaffolding; they provided the experience of life with schizophrenia and the knowledge of the mental health system. Among us, we had the expertise we needed to carry out the research.

Underlying this discussion of levels of service user involvement in research is the central issue of power. The success of service user involvement in research depends on an awareness of power differentials and a willingness on the part of professional researchers to share power.[5] However, one cannot simply 'give' people power; they must also be willing and ready to take it up. I came to our research with academic training, professional status, and research experience, attributes likely to offer me significantly more access to power than people without these attributes. The members of the research group were self-selected – anyone in the Unsung Heroes support group who wanted to take part was welcome. They came with no experience of doing research, only their experiences of being research subjects and their experiences in the mental health system, which had taught them to be passive recipients of services and to expect to have very little control over most aspects of their lives. They began the research with 'trepidation and uncertainty,' as Michele said, about the whole enterprise. They did not, at first, think of themselves as experts in anything. Their roles in the research changed during the course of the project as they became more confident and realized that they were in fact quite able to make decisions and suggest next steps.

Fisher's ideas about communication as uncoerced, mutual, educative exchange point to the attitude and approach necessary for negotiating these power issues. But putting his ideas about communication into practice was harder than it sounds. Finding a balance between keeping the research going and not being too bossy was for me the most challenging aspect of the projects. I worried constantly about my role in the process. Was I being too directive, or not directive enough? Was I pushing them too hard, or not enough? Was I expecting too much of them and myself? Was I listening to them carefully enough? I never really had a sense that I knew what we were or should be doing, and as the academic member of the group, I was the one who was supposed to know this! I learned to let go of my need to be in control and to appreciate the unfolding of the process as the group members learned to take more control and direct this unfolding. An excerpt from my journal gives a sense of my uncertainty.

> *Barbara's Journal, 15 January 2002. On the very first day of the project, Dana suggested that what I was really doing was testing them to see if they could do the task. Paranoia, or just too much experience of the mental health system where they are continually tested to see what they can and cannot do? My reaction was shock that they would think this, followed by the thought that I could be doing that too. The boundaries in PAR are clearly problematic.*

In one significant way I retained control in both projects. Our proposals for funding were successful because of the kind of research we proposed to do, but also, at least in part, because of my record of previous grants and academic publications. Following a long tradition for granting agencies, they awarded the grants to me, the professional researcher. The SSHRC grant required that it be administered by my university and that we hire graduate students as research assistants. Granting agencies quite reasonably seek to ensure both professional competence in the conduct of the research and accountability in the spending of the money. If this had been a truly user-controlled project, the grants would have been awarded to the group and they would have had control over how the money was spent and who was hired to help. Instead the money remained under my control, and although we discussed as a group how some of it would be spent, I also spent money on various aspects of the projects without consulting them. If granting agencies see the value of involving service recipients in research, they may in the future want to reconsider how some grants are awarded and administered. This might mean including service users on adjudication committees and awarding money to groups that do not have institutional affiliations.

What We Did

The following description of our projects makes it sound as if we knew exactly what we were doing and moved smoothly from one phase of the research to the next. This was not the case. I began the first project with no real idea of what to expect. I had to learn what the various members of the group could and couldn't do and to organize the work around their abilities. It took me a while to realize that all the work had to happen in the meetings. We had to deal with side conversations, keep people on topic, and negotiate different interests in the group. But this is not really different from any situation in which a group of people undertakes a complicated project. The doubts, frustrations, and uncertainties I experienced in the project were similar to those I have experienced in all the research projects I have undertaken. Where will we find people to interview? Can we get agencies to help us? What should we do next? Do we have any idea of what we are doing? Will this project turn out to be worthwhile? We stumbled along, making our decisions on the basis of what we thought might work best or what was actually doable under the circumstances, learning as we went. Some meetings were very productive, others not so productive. In all, it was a very intense experience and at several points in the projects we took breaks, cancelling a meeting or two to give everyone a breather. Now that we have accomplished something we are all proud of, even we sometimes look back and think we knew what we were doing. The rosy glow of memory has obscured all the uncertainties and doubts we experienced.

Getting Ethics Approval

Ethics approval for both research projects was obtained from the University of Calgary Research Ethics Board. The board at that time was unfamiliar with participatory research, especially involving what they regarded as a 'vulnerable population.' I was fortunate that the chair of the board was one of my colleagues – her office was down the hall from mine – so I had the opportunity to talk with her at some length about the project. We discussed the rationale for carrying out the research in the way that we proposed and what the research would ask of the people taking part. I had carried out a number of research projects using a variety of qualitative methods, and although in participatory research it is impossible to predict exactly how a project will unfold, I had a strong sense of what I thought the Unsung Heroes could achieve. This discussion smoothed the way to speedy approval of the project. In our second project, Michele (the coordinator of the Unsung Heroes Peer Support Group) and I were summoned to meet with the full board, who again were worried about the 'vulnerable population,' and about the fact that this time we proposed to use visual methods, including a photo collage and a video, to disseminate the research. Having completed the first project, both Michele and I now knew exactly what would be asked of the people taking part. Michele did most of the talking, clearly rejecting what she regarded as the paternalistic concerns of the board, stressing that group members had initiated the second project because of their experience in the first, that they were eager to take part, and that they objected to being regarded as vulnerable or as too dim-witted to decide for themselves whether to take part. In fact, their inclusion as full researchers would help to accomplish the goal of the ethics committee to ensure the protection of others like themselves from exploitation or coercion. Board approval was forthcoming, with the proviso that we show all of our visual materials to the board chair before dissemination to ensure that we were not putting the participants in jeopardy or exposing them by revealing their identities in problematic ways.

All the members of the research group (including me and the graduate student research assistants) signed consent forms, and, when others were interviewed, they also signed consent forms. Our professional transcriber signed a confidentiality form. Members of the research group were not offered confidentiality or anonymity, as it was the intention from the beginning of the projects that co-researchers who wanted to would take part in the dissemination of the research. Interviewees from outside the group were offered confidentiality and anonymity; in order to preserve their anonymity, no names are associated with the quotations from the interviews that appear in the next two chapters.

The First Project

In September of 2001, Michele, the coordinator of the Unsung Heroes group, invited anyone who was interested to attend the first meeting of the research group. I no longer remember how many people attended this meeting, and attendance was variable throughout the course of the research, but a core group of seven members became engaged in the first project. Meetings took place twice a month from 5:30 to 6:30, right before the regular 7:00 p.m. Unsung Heroes support group meetings, so that group members would not have to make an extra trip to the Schizophrenia Society. All group members were paid for their participation at a rate of $8.00 per hour (including time for travel as well as meeting time), and people from outside the group received an honorarium of a $25 grocery store gift card for taking part in their interview.

CHOOSING THE TOPIC

In our first meeting, we began by brainstorming a number of topics that group members were interested in investigating. Among other topics, they articulated a vague goal of investigating what they called 'stigma' among their medical professionals. They were concerned about the subtle and not so subtle ways in which they experience rudeness, dismissiveness, and outright discrimination both in hospital and in their outpatient interactions. They had a strong sense that what they experience in their treatment relationships is different from what people with other illnesses experience and they wanted to do something to change this. We settled on this topic as something that was of interest to everyone. At the time, we simply asked: What are the experiences of people diagnosed with schizophrenia in the mental health system? We later came to call this communication with medical professionals, but the idea that we could tie what we were interested in to communication did not emerge until quite late in the analysis stage of the project.

DESIGNING THE RESEARCH

After settling on the topic and research question, we considered a number of methods for doing the research. Group members really knew of only one method – surveys. I described a range of other methods, including in-depth one-on-one interviews, focus groups (which are really group interviews), and ethnography (which involves studying social settings by observing them, either as a participant or as an outsider). The idea that they could talk directly to their colleagues about their experiences was very exciting to the group and they decided to conduct in-depth interviews. One of the group members suggested that we construct a list of interview questions that we could use to get interviewees talking about the right kinds of things. We brainstormed questions, with each member contributing ideas that he or she thought were relevant to the research topic. These included such things as when and how the person came to be diagnosed with schizophrenia, what their hospital experiences had been like, who had been most helpful to them in adjusting to life with schizophrenia, and how they had found the strategies they used to cope with having schizophrenia. I took notes and organized the questions into groups of related questions. At the next meeting, the group went over the list, revising, adding, or deleting as seemed appropriate. After the questions were finalized, a copy was printed for each member of the group. (See appendix A for the lists of questions in both projects.)

DOING THE INTERVIEWS

Interviews began in January of 2002. We decided to start by doing interviews among the members of our immediate group. Except for me, none of the members of the group had ever conducted interviews and most had never been interviewed. All were quite nervous, questioning their ability both to conduct interviews and to be interviewed. But as with every stage of the research process, group members learned by doing. We had a meeting at which we discussed what was entailed in interviewing. I asked them for their suggestions on how to conduct a 'good' interview. They talked about eye contact, tone of voice, listening, not interrupting, nodding sympathetically, asking follow-up questions, and so on. As a group they knew everything they needed to know about how to carry out an interview. Two brave people then offered to be the first to interview and be interviewed. This was followed by more group discussion of what they thought worked well in this interview and how the next pair might improve upon what had been done.

All interviews took place in the group setting. We sat around the table in the Schizophrenia Society office meeting room, with a little digital audio recorder sitting on the table, while one member of the group interviewed another member. There was some anxiety about the audio recorder, but they soon got used to that. During the first interview, after the interviewer had asked her first question, the man being interviewed turned to me and said something like, 'Do I get a list of answers to choose from?' He had experience only with surveys in which his responses were limited to those identified as possibilities by the researcher. Once the group members realized that they were free to say whatever they wanted in their answers, they never looked back. As the interviews proceeded, all members of the group took part, either as interviewers, interviewees, or both, and their confidence in their ability to participate in the process increased. We also conducted interviews with a few people who attended Unsung Heroes meetings sporadically and came to the research group meeting only to be interviewed. The journal entries give an idea of our experiences in the first few interviews:

Barbara's Journal, 11 January 2002. Hearing [group member] talk – I had hardly heard his voice before today. But he was articulate, confident, sure of what he had to say. You could hear a pin drop. Everyone was there, completely attentive.
Laurie's Journal, 17 January 2002. I was asked to do an interview but I felt a little nervous. Maybe later I will. I do feel free to talk and make comments about topics and interviews.

Dana's Journal, 7 February 2002. We are on our way. George and Mark inter-view very concise and to the point. Direct questions and to-the-point answers. Mark did very well in answering the questions. He was very clear, and he had good insight into many aspects of the illness. It makes him feel weighted down, like walking in slavery. George asked questions on an even note, no highs or lows, and a nice friendly voice for questions.

As time passed, the group members became fully engaged in the re-search process and everyone became very comfortable with the experi-ence of interviewing. The people who had not yet been interviewed looked forward to their chance to talk about themselves, and the oth-ers looked forward to hearing their stories. We fell into a pattern of conducting two interviews at each meeting, each about half an hour long. Interviewers became much more comfortable following lines of questioning, rather than sticking to the questions on the list, and those who were listening felt free to jump in to the interview if they heard something they wanted to follow up on. We conducted the final inter-views as group interviews: one person agreed to be interviewed, but no one was designated as the interviewer, and anyone who wanted to ask questions did so. As the interviews progressed, we realized that we had created a space in which group members could talk freely about aspects of their lives that they normally have no opportunity to talk about. The Unsung Heroes meetings provide some opportunity to talk about past experiences, but the primary purpose is dealing with current problems. Hearing details of the life experiences of group members was often emotional, both for those who were describing their experiences and for those who were listening. The structure of the interview process allowed even people who rarely spoke in our meetings to tell their stories. Through the interviewing, we became a caring and supportive community of friends. Laurie's journal entries give a sense of her expe-rience as an interviewer and as a listener:

Laurie's Journal, 7 February 2002. It was great listening to Mark. Usually he doesn't say too much. He put into words what I think a lot of us feel when living with the illness. Knowing you are not alone is so important.
Laurie's Journal, 7 February 2002. I really feel different doing the interview. I was so interested in what Michele was saying that I lost track of the questions I was asking.
Laurie's Journal, 21 February 2002. I did another interview asking George questions. I found again it was interesting listening to answers. I tried to ask

more in the same line, so he would explain more fully. What amazes me is most people remember the medications they were on over the years, which can be a lot. It seems to me a lot of the medications have long difficult names and lots of side effects, and most remember what the side effects are.

ANALYSING THE DATA

The interviews concluded in April of 2002, and in May we began data analysis. We had eleven interview transcripts and one transcript of an earlier group discussion in which group members had talked generally about their treatment experiences both in and out of hospital. These transcripts were made from the tape recordings by a professional transcriber. The group members, without any input from me (I was in another room photocopying the transcripts at the time they had this conversation), decided to conduct a thematic analysis of the data, although they did not call it that. That is, based on the experience of listening to the interviews, they had a strong intuitive sense that they wanted to compare people's stories on a number of topics that everyone seemed to have mentioned. These included such topics as the numerous medications people had taken over the years, the various diagnoses they had received, their interactions with doctors and nurses, and their good and bad experiences in hospitals. They thought that they could come up with a list of categories, assign a colour to each category, and use coloured highlighters to code the transcripts, although they did not use this 'research methods' vocabulary to describe the process.

We then began coding the transcripts, reading them and marking sections with the appropriate colours to indicate the topics that were talked about in those sections. Group members had great difficulty with this part of the research process. Their journal entries give a sense of the challenges of reading the transcripts and also a sense of the emotional impact of reading their own transcripts:

Dana's Journal, 16 May 2002. I really don't like trying to figure out what is good, bad, or indifferent about the things I have read in these papers. I prefer not to categorize it and let someone else do it. It's hard to tell if my feelings for something would be the same as someone else's. I would just like to get on with the writing of the presentation.
Laurie's Journal, 16 May 2002. I read the transcript of my interview. I had trouble believing I talked like this. I realized a while ago that I have a communication problem, but I didn't realize it was this bad. I think what I'm going to say, but when I go to speak, it doesn't come out the same. A lot of the time I can't

pronounce the words or haven't finished a sentence. I repeat words, and say words I didn't mean to say. No wonder people have trouble understanding me and look at me with blank looks sometimes.

After two meetings at which we made almost no progress in coding the transcripts, Hannah Scissons, a graduate student in communications studies from the University of Calgary, was hired to assist with the data analysis. She used the categories that group members had created – medications, support, diagnosis, good experiences, bad experiences – and added the central category of communication in which all the others were embedded. She proposed an analytic scheme that incorporated all of the categories using the idea of good and bad experiences to frame the analysis (see figure 1). She then presented this scheme to the group members for discussion. They were very taken with her diagram. They could immediately see the relationships between their original categories and were impressed with the way a diagram could present the essence of their stories in such a coherent way. After some discussion and a few modifications, this diagram was used to organize the results that are presented in chapter 3. Here is my journal entry for the meeting at which Hannah presented the analytic scheme:

> **Barbara's Journal, 6 June 2002.** *Hannah showed her chart and then quickly in a few sentences explained how it all fitted together. The whole thing came to life as she talked – and everyone felt it do so. A very exciting experience.*

The Second Project

In our second project on housing for people diagnosed with schizophrenia, we followed a very similar pattern. The topic had been chosen by the group members at the end of the first project. I wrote the grant application and revised it based on input mainly from Michele but also from the person who was then executive director of Schizophrenia Society. After we got the grant, Michele invited anyone in the Unsung Heroes who was interested to attend the first meeting of the project. I had prepared an information sheet that described what we would be doing and told potential group members that the project would take two years. If people were interested in taking part, I asked them to sign this sheet to indicate they understood the time commitment required. We again met twice a month for an hour before the regular Unsung Heroes meetings starting in April of 2005. The group included four

Figure 1. Hannah's Diagram: Communication with Medical Professionals

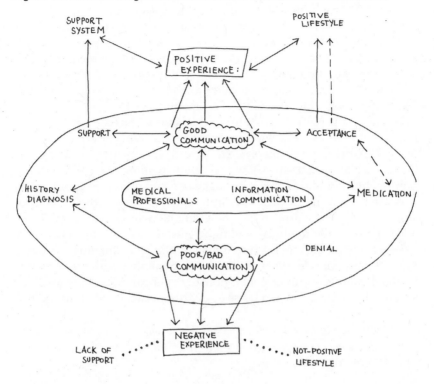

people who had taken part in the first project and five new members. All were paid $9 per hour for their participation, including, meetings, travel time, interviews, focus groups, presentations, and anything else we did. Participants from outside the group again received a $25 grocery store gift card.

DESIGNING THE RESEARCH
We used our first meetings to discuss our goals and to decide on the procedures for carrying out the research. Group members wanted to talk about housing experiences with people who have schizophrenia and have experienced homelessness or housing instability. As in the first project, they wanted to do in-depth interviews, and this time they also wanted to conduct some focus groups. After much discussion, we decided that we would ask interviewees to self-identify as people liv-

ing with schizophrenia rather than asking for medical evidence that they had schizophrenia. We again spent several meetings generating a list of questions to ask in the interviews and focus groups. This time the focus of the questions was on how people came to lose their housing, what it was like not having stable housing, who had helped them find stable housing, and how they maintained their housing stability. Laurie proposed a question that we wanted to be sure we asked each person: 'What does home mean to you?' (See appendix A.)

We came up with a list of individuals and housing agencies who might help us to find people to interview. Having been around the mental health and housing systems in Calgary for many years, group members had a good sense of who might be willing to help. I made appointments with the people they suggested and one of the group members went with me to each appointment. We asked if they would be able to connect us with people who might be willing to be interviewed and whether they might be willing to host a focus group. They were very supportive and sounded as if they would be willing to help, but in the end it became clear that most were just too busy and overwhelmed by the demands of running their housing agencies to become involved with us. My journal gives a sense of my discouragement at this point:

Barbara's Journal, 5 July 2005. *We seem to have come to a complete halt in our research. I don't know how aggressively to harass the agencies, who are actually too busy to focus on helping us.*

Group members suggested that they could ask the agencies they were connected to if they could put up recruitment notices, so lots of our pink notices appeared in places that are frequented by people diagnosed with schizophrenia. We were also greatly assisted by Potential Place Clubhouse, where we found quite a number of people to interview. Laurie and I visited her therapist, who expressed a willingness to send people to us.[6] In all of our recruitment, we were challenged by our (very reasonable) agreement with the ethics committee that agency employees and other professionals could not give us the names and contact information of potential interviewees. Instead they passed on our contact information and we had to wait for people to call us. A few people did in fact call us, but not very many. Instead we found most of our interviewees through personal contacts of group members. Two agencies did finally agree to host focus groups, for which we were very grateful.

DOING THE INTERVIEWS AND FOCUS GROUPS

In our first project, most of the interviewing had taken place within the group. As we were going further afield this time, we felt a need to be better prepared. We invited a guest from the sociology department at the University of Calgary, Liza McCoy, to come to one of our meetings and talk to us about conducting interviews and focus groups. We ran this very informally with Liza simply responding to questions from group members. Should we assign specific group members to ask specific questions? Do we have to stick to the order of our pre-planned questions? What do you do when you lose your train of thought? What if we run out of questions? Should we ask each person in a focus group to answer each question? How do we get quiet people to talk more? She helped us to feel confident that we could really do a good job of this. One piece of advice that we took up with enthusiasm was her suggestion to provide 'quiet' food, so that eating noises would not interfere with our tape recording. We settled on mini-muffins available at a convenient grocery store as our perfect interview and focus group food. Laurie describes what she learned from Liza's visit:

Laurie's Journal, 15 September 2005. Liza McCoy from the University of Calgary Sociology department came to talk to us about how to do group interviews. She answered all our questions. Something Liza suggested that I found helpful was that it is really important to try and let focus group members have a dialogue about their situations, to encourage them to talk about something they have in common. What are the barriers they have or problems they have getting good housing? Have them compare stories, ask them questions like 'did they find an organization helpful or not?' It is more listening and directing the conversation when needed. To think of areas of conversations as doorways that have to be opened. To remember if you have four good topics to introduce you can't go too wrong.

We again began by conducting interviews among the group members. These interviews provided a safe environment for group members to practise interviewing as well as a way to generate data. After we had conducted a few interviews, we had a workshop night at which group members identified specific interview strategies that they felt enhanced or impeded the interviews. We practised the helpful strategies and critiqued each other. Several group members became extremely skilled interviewers over the course of the project.

At this time, I used some of our grant money to purchase video equipment for the project. We hoped to make a video at the end of the project and wanted to begin recording our meetings and interviews for use in it. Tom Everrett, a graduate student from the Faculty of Communication and Culture who later made our documentary film, trained Dale, the most technically savvy group member, to use the camera and to make good recordings. Dale brought the camera to meetings and interviews and videotaped the proceedings. Anyone who was not comfortable being videotaped was seated out of range of the camera. Cindy's journal describes her experience of being filmed:

> *Cindy's Journal, 16 June 2005. I was taped last week. It was a lot of fun to see myself on the little camera and hear myself. I was a little nervous.*

We were now ready to ask people from outside the group to come to our meetings to be interviewed. Typically, two group members acted as the primary interviewers, but others felt free to jump in if they had something they wanted to ask. The interviewee and the interviewers were seated together at one side of the room and other group members were seated around the room. We also interviewed people from outside the group in a variety of locations, including in their homes, in coffee shops, and in a room provided by an agency that had connected us with them. One or two members of the research group (sometimes more) and I attended each of these interviews. The journal entries show how group members experienced the interviews:

> *Laurie's Journal, 12 May 2005. Rachel's (not her real name) story. When interviewing Rachel I found it difficult to go on asking questions when she told of the abuse she had to endure, starting with her childhood, and of being a homeless person for fourteen years. How she endured it is hard for me to understand. It took one caring person who had the contacts to get Rachel the help she needed.*
>
> *George's Journal, 12 May 2005. Today we interviewed Rachel. She left home because she was abused physically and mentally. A minister in the Catholic church gave her money for one night in a hotel. She was on the street on and off for fourteen years. She tried to commit suicide, and she traded sex for housing.*
>
> *Laurie's Journal, September 2005. Interview experience with Leslie (not her real name). I didn't realize how hard interviewing would be at times. The case in point is when trying to interview Leslie about her experience of being homeless. We realized Leslie was not well. It is a relief to know Leslie is now in a stable housing situation. Leslie has good supports to help her manage her medication. What Leslie most wanted was for the symptoms of illness to stop. It is hard to imagine someone coping with schizophrenia while being homeless. It is so troubling inter-*

*viewing a person who is struggling with the illness, even when they have a home
and supports in place.*

Laurie's Journal, 6 October 2005. *Interview with Veronika (not her real name).
Michele and I interviewed Veronika. She was released from the hospital with no
medication, no phone call was made to family or friends before she was released.
She had no home to go to at the time. Fortunately, after a number of days on the
streets she found her way to her sister's home, who took her in and gave her shelter. Her sister was a great support for her.*

Laurie's Journal, 25 November 2005. *Interview with James (not his real name).
James spent a lot of his hardest times in Edmonton. He had hospitalizations, homeless periods, and talked about the rougher side of life. He explained that most of his
homeless times were when he stopped taking his medication. He also mentioned
how in the 1980s and around that time, the side effects from the medications were
much more difficult to cope with. He finds the medications available now are so
much better. He is someone who would like to help others. He ended the interview
by letting Dr Barbara Schneider and me know how he found talking to us such a
positive experience.*

Over about eight months, we interviewed twenty individuals, including eight members of the research group and twelve from outside
the group. We also conducted two focus groups with people outside
the group. One of these groups consisted of five people from outside
the group and three interviewers from the group. The other consisted
of eleven people from outside the group (some of whom observed but
did not participate) and five interviewers from the group. Group members regarded these focus groups as highlights of the interviewing por-
tion of the project. They felt they were hearing from people they would
never otherwise have had the opportunity to talk to about issues of real
importance to all of them. Laurie describes one of these focus groups:

Laurie's Journal, 13 October 2005. *Focus Group at the Mustard Seed. We met
with a group of ten to fifteen people at the Mustard Seed who chose to talk to us
about their housing situation. We selected five questions; Dr Barbara Schneider,
Claude, Cindy, Michele, Mary, and I took turns asking each member in the focus
group a question. I was asked to start. When I asked my question I found eye
contact very important and to really listen to each person. People diagnosed with
schizophrenia have a lot of common problems. Having difficulty being compliant
to the mental health system. Learning what organizations and help were available
and how to access them. Managing and having enough money. Also keeping well
enough to manage their financial affairs. Family support was very important. A*

lot of the times the help forthcoming wasn't very tangible – i.e. 'The most help I ever received was from [agency name]. They gave me money for my damage deposit and first month's rent for my apartment.' As the interviewing continued the dialogue opened up and participants felt more comfortable with the process. The people taking part said it meant a lot to them to participate and they hoped this research project could make a difference to the homeless situation.

ANALYSING THE DATA

All interviews and focus groups were audio-recorded and transcribed by our professional transcriber. Copies of all the transcripts were then given to the research group members to read. Except for me, no one in the research group had attended every interview and focus group. Although not every group member read the approximately four hundred pages of transcripts, those who did found that doing so gave them access to everything that had taken place in the project up to that time. The members who read the transcripts wrote a summary of what they felt were the main themes and important ideas in the interviews. In her journal, Laurie comments on her reading of the transcripts:

Laurie's Journal, 24 February 2006. Transcripts. I finally managed to read through all the transcripts of the interviews that the research group has done to date. I could not quite believe the massive amount of material there was to read. It took over a week for me to read through it all. I tried to make notes as I went along. Mary and Michele have covered most of the key points in their reports. I went ahead doing the best I could, realizing my report might contribute to emphasizing recurring themes.

The analytic focus for the results developed as we explored various themes and ideas in our meetings, looking for a way to organize our data that would reflect the experiences of the group members and of the people we had interviewed. At one particularly dynamic meeting, we discussed the difficulties of being long-term care recipients, something that resonated deeply with all the members of the group. This meeting generated a tremendous outpouring of emotion as group members articulated their experiences of being caught in what we came to call the dilemmas of care and control. This idea became the focus of the analysis. Transcripts were given to a research assistant who coded them using HyperResearch, a computer program for qualitative data analysis. I used this coding to identify key sections of the data for inclusion in the results presented in chapter 4.

NOT JUST A RESEARCH PROJECT

We didn't work all the time. At one of our early meetings in the housing project, we carried out an activity that promoted a sense of belonging and encouraged our friendships to flourish. Monique Solomon, one of the graduate research assistants, suggested and led this activity. We wanted to write short biographies of the group members, so Monique asked the group as a whole to generate a description of each member. Each person had a turn at listening to the others' descriptions of them. They heard themselves described along a range of personal characteristics such as having a good sense of humour or being reliable, generous, and logical. They also heard themselves described in terms of the skills and abilities that each brought to the project such as being a good listener, a good interviewer, or a supportive group member. Each person, including Monique and me, experienced the power of being seen as valuable and worthy in the eyes of others. I suspect that this is a standard kind of team-building exercise used in many settings, although I had never taken part in such an exercise before. I can speak only for myself about the wonderful feeling this experience produced in me of being regarded as an important member of the group. For each person, it provided strong evidence that the others thought of him or her as a valuable and contributing member with many positive personal characteristics.

Monique and Laurie suggested and organized an art and writing session for the group. Laurie is a practising artist and runs an art group for the Schizophrenia Society. She organized all the materials she thought we would need, including paper and various drawing and painting media. The pictures we produced can be seen on our project website. Monique brought a sheet for group members to write about themselves and why they were involved in the project. This was a very successful session. Laurie describes:

Laurie's Journal, 17 November 2005. Art and Writing Night. Tonight we were to draw 'What Home Means to Me.' It was a night of fun. My daughter Amy came to help out. The group members were to draw and colour a picture of what home means to them. Amy and I brainstormed some ideas of what would help them start to draw. We started with a circle as a starting point and encouraged people to express themselves in any way they felt comfortable. If they didn't know where to start, we had them think of home, what comes to mind. Some people chose to be more abstract. We asked them to write a few words about what they had drawn. Jamal helped with the writing.

We also had a number of group dinners. Laurie describes two of these:

> **Laurie's Journal, 14 December 2005.** *Christmas Dinner. It was great for all of us to get together for supper. I found I got to chat with everyone about day-to-day things. I enjoyed saying hello to everyone and wishing everyone well for the holidays. It was lots of fun, everyone seemed happy, and it was great just socializing. I felt relaxed, where sometimes in restaurants I am nervous. I am looking forward to the new year and being part of the group again.*
>
> **Laurie's Journal, 23 December 2006.** *We all met at the Silver Dragon at noon for a Christmas get-together. It was my first time having Dim Sum and for most of the rest of the group it was a new experience. I was closest to where the carts went by, so I was in charge of ordering. I had to ask what most of the food items were. They all tasted so good and the rest of group seemed to enjoy the food too. It went fast. We had fun talking and sharing. It was a good time.*

At one of our data analysis meetings, group members discussed their experiences of being on the disability pension in Alberta, Assured Income for the Severely Handicapped (AISH), which all but one of them are on. They had some uncertainties about changes that had been recently implemented in the program and what they were actually entitled to. Laurie's journal conveys some of the discussion:

> **Laurie's Journal, 6 January 2007.** *We spent time talking about a recurring topic that came up during interviewing. AISH was something that seemed to have an incredible impact on most of us. Having the stable income gave us food, clothing, shelter, and medicine. But for a lot of us the stress of having to follow all of AISH rules and requirements made living harsh and created a lot of fear. Especially when we have workers who have differing requirements. Also because of the overwhelming paperwork that we have to complete to receive our AISH. Workers are not responsible for their mistakes, their clients are, which can result in a client suffering financially for their worker's mistakes. Plus rules can change from worker to worker. At this meeting it was interesting listening to others and realizing it was a highly emotional topic. Most had a lot of fear around AISH.*

We invited an administrator from AISH to come to one of our meetings to answer questions about how AISH works. The meeting did answer some questions, but for me the real value of the meeting was in demonstrating the appropriateness of the approach that we had chosen for carrying out our research. Community-based participatory action research[7] is becoming an increasingly popular approach to the involvement of community members in research. It brings together people from a variety of diverse stakeholder groups to research a problem of concern to them all – for example, mental health care workers, administrators, service recipients, and professional researchers. Taking this broader approach might have helped us, particularly in the dissemination phase of the projects, but the behaviour and attitude of the group members during the meeting with the AISH administrator showed me why it was important for our project not to involve anyone who might be seen by the group members as an authority figure. They immediately became polite, deferential, and accommodating. They did have a chance to air some of their grievances with the pension system, but mainly they listened politely as the administrator explained how busy and overworked her staff were and how much trouble they were having adapting to the changes in the system. While this is the organizational context within which the experiences of people diagnosed with schizophrenia unfold, it also dramatically illustrated for me how the years of dealing with authority figures in the mental health system have affected their willingness to assert themselves in the presence of those they perceive as having control over their lives. In fact I saw a demonstration of how people diagnosed with schizophrenia negotiate the dilemmas of care and control that we take up in our discussions in the next two chapters.

3 What We Learned: Communication between People Diagnosed with Schizophrenia and Their Medical Professionals (Results)

WITH HANNAH SCISSONS

'For cancer or heart attacks or anything they always tell you, "You've had a heart attack, you've got cancer, you've got leukemia." Only with mental illnesses they won't tell us.' —Michele Misurelli

'A lot of the psychiatrists today, they treat you as if they have learned from the previous patient. They don't really treat you as an individual. They treat the illness, not the person you used to be a long time ago.' —George Benson

In this chapter and the next, I present the stories of the people who were interviewed for our projects. The results from the two projects are interrelated, but because the projects were done at different times with different groups of co-researchers, I present them in separate chapters. Chapter 3 addresses the interaction between people diagnosed with schizophrenia and their medical professionals, focusing on the kind of communication that is needed to improve this relationship. Good medical treatment is, however, only one aspect of what is necessary for people to rebuild satisfying lives. Chapter 4 therefore broadens the discussion to examine a nexus of factors that combine to promote stability in the lives of people diagnosed with schizophrenia, focused around the central topic of how people achieve stable housing. At the end of each chapter are recommendations that group members generated for their service providers.

Chapter 4 takes up a thread that is implicit but not articulated in our discussion of communication in chapter 3 – the hidden and frequently not-so-hidden undercurrent of control that seems to be inherent in the care that is provided to people diagnosed with schizophrenia. This tension between care and control produces dilemmas for people diagnosed with schizophrenia that they must negotiate in all their interactions with their service providers. Here it becomes clear that inclusion as partners in decision-making about their own treatment and housing, achieved through communication, is the key to mitigating this control and to reducing the burden of these dilemmas. Inclusion in decision-making enables people diagnosed with schizophrenia to recover a sense of themselves as people who can live both 'within and beyond'[1] the diagnosis of schizophrenia.

Although participants in our projects describe many negative experiences with the medical and housing systems, our research is offered not so much to be critical as to increase understanding of the experiences of people diagnosed with schizophrenia. We do not speak for all people diagnosed with schizophrenia, only for the people who were interviewed for these projects. What follows represents the words, experiences, and thoughts of these people as understood and interpreted by the members of our research groups.

Results

The results in our first project are organized around four main interrelated themes of diagnosis, medications, information/support, and interaction, all of which are embedded in the central issue of communication. Two aspects of communication – communication as the capacity to transfer information and communication as the ability to build relationships – are relevant in understanding the experiences of the people interviewed for this project. Also relevant are Fisher's ideas about communication, in which each party responds to and learns from the other. As Fisher describes, the ideal communicative interaction offers 'equal opportunity to participate, to criticize, to express personal aims and attitudes, and to perform these acts without regard to power or ideology.'[2] Persuasion of both parties, each by the other, is an inevitable consequence of communication that honours the dignity and worth of all participants. The goal is not only mutual understanding but also 'practical wisdom and humane action.'[3] Fisher's understanding of communication does not describe the traditional doctor-patient relationship, particularly the paternalistic treatment of people diagnosed with schizophrenia discussed in chapter 1. His ideas offer instead the understanding that people diagnosed with schizophrenia as well as medical practitioners have legitimate perspectives that must be acknowledged and integrated in the treatment relationship.

When the people who were interviewed were not told their diagnosis, were not given adequate information about medications and their side effects, were not informed about schizophrenia and where they could find support, and were not treated with dignity and respect, they generally had bad experiences with medical professionals and stayed in a state of denial about having schizophrenia. When information was more successfully communicated to them, when the diagnosis was clear, the medications explained, support made available, and their concerns heard, and when they were treated with dignity and respect, they generally had more positive experiences with medical professionals. They began to accept that they were ill, come to terms with having schizophrenia, and learn to live with and beyond their diagnosis.

Diagnosis

Diagnosis can be problematic in mental health, and it is often very hard for medical practitioners to come to a definitive diagnosis. But when doctors are reluctant to commit themselves to a specific diagnosis, when the diagnosis takes years to come to or changes frequently, or when people are simply not told anything specific, it is extremely distressing for them. This lack of clear definition about the nature of their situation is very frustrating and can make it much harder for people to adjust. One person described receiving mixed messages from her doctors: 'When I first went to the hospital, my doctor did not tell me. The practising student doctor took me aside, and he says, "We think you have paranoid schizophrenia." But my doctor would not tell me. He did not give me the diagnosis.'

A number of the participants talked about a time when their diagnosis became clear to them. Before that time they remember trying to understand conflicting diagnoses and feeling confused and frustrated in their interactions with their doctors. Many participants described a long period when they and their doctors did not know what was wrong. One participant noted that it took almost fourteen years for doctors to diagnose his disorder. Another still has not received a clear diagnosis from her doctors. She feels that knowing her diagnosis is essential in order to be able to deal with having a mental illness. Many have had a number of doctors over the years, each giving a different diagnosis. As one woman said, 'First it was schizophrenia, then manic depression, then hypo something, hypo activity or some type of thing. Then another one was that I had no adolescence. And then the last one was schizo-affective. So, what really does the diagnosis mean?' Another participant told of his frustration with a change in his diagnosis on the very day of the interview for this project, saying, 'I was told today that my diagnosis with schizophrenia seven years ago may be flawed. I feel like I'm living a big lie. I'm fed up with it and I wish that some big fool would make up their mind.' Without a clear diagnosis, participants could not begin to deal with having schizophrenia. And even with a clear diagnosis, being labelled is in itself problematic. As one man said, 'You have to be labelled, and that was the hardest thing. It was like, "Oh man, this is all I need."'

Medications

Participants reported that in addition to a lack of information from medical professionals about diagnosis, there was also a lack of information about the antipsychotic medications used for treatment. These medications are a central reality in the lives of people diagnosed with schizophrenia, and they can be quite effective for many (but certainly not all) in controlling the experiences of hallucinations and delusions. These medications also produce an array of sometimes debilitating side effects. The participants talked often and at length about their experiences with different medications. The trade-off that is clear for medical professionals – that it is better to take medication to reduce psychotic symptoms and put up with severe side effects – is not at all so clear to those who have to take the medications.

Many noted the unwillingness of their doctors to discuss treatment options with them. They complained about not being able to communicate their experiences with and concerns about medications, particularly the debilitating side effects of the medications. In fact, they were often not informed at all by their doctors about possible side effects. As one person said, 'They don't tell you about the side effects, and the side effects are just incredible.' Another described how the medications were presented to her:

They just said, 'You have to take your choice; you either take the meds and take the repercussions, which are the side effects, or you go around being insane. So what do you want to do? You have to pick.' Do I want to walk around crazy, or do I take weight gain and stiffness and blurred vision and dry mouth and all the other things? They just kind of forced it and said, 'You have to take this.' There was just no argument with them. They were saying this works.

One participant said he was not told about possible changes in his mental state when he changed from one medication to another: 'I'm really going to give it to [my doctor] with both barrels, because I changed over to Olanzapine [an antipsychotic medication] and he didn't tell me it would take two weeks to kick in properly.' Another recounted her doctor's dismissal of her concern about the weight gain caused by her medication:

> I was concerned about my weight gain...and I'm bringing up this concern, and he says, 'Well, don't you feel more voluptuous? Don't you notice men noticing you more?' And I'm like, 'What?' I said, 'What is wrong with you? I don't feel that way. Actually I feel less attractive and I don't feel healthy.'

Many described what they felt was overmedication at various stages of their medical treatment. As one person said, 'The meds totally zonked me out, because my doctor medicated me to the ying-yang. I was a walking zombie. Somebody would ask me something, I'd go, "Whaaat?" That was the worst time.' One person said that he mistook the side effects of the medication for the symptoms of the illness. Another talked about a time when the side effects were so bad that he decided to go off his medications. As another person said, 'It is really hard to explain to them how it feels when they give us too much, but it is like being tied up in certain areas of us.' One man's description of being on medication struck a particular chord among the research group members: 'I feel weighted down by the medication. It's hard to move, walk, do things. It's like walking in slavery, like lifting heavy bricks all the time, weighed down by the illness.'

Information and Support

Receiving information about schizophrenia and about where they can get support is essential for people to be able to cope with having schizophrenia. Even when the diagnosis is a definite one, there is no guarantee that it will actually be 'clear' to the person. As one person said, he had little comprehension of what schizophrenia was when he was first told he had it, and as a result he experienced fear and apprehension. Participants recalled their doctors being less helpful in providing information than nurses, who were often instrumental in steering them to support groups such as the Schizophrenia Society. Some participants sought out information on their own from places such as the internet. One woman recounted finding out about a source of support quite accidentally: 'I was totally ignorant about schizophrenia. And then one day I was watching television, and there was a little blurb about volunteer places. I saw this little ad for the Schizophrenia Society, and I said, "Oh, I never heard of that place." I wrote down the phone number and I called.' Participants also emphasized that they want their doctors to communicate with family and friends and to provide them with information about schizophrenia. If family members do not understand what they are experiencing, it is difficult if not impossible for them to be sources of support.

Many participants described themselves as being in denial, especially when they were first diagnosed, and said that they were not told that they were ill or given any information that would help them overcome the denial. Participants acknowledge that when they are in the grip of psychosis, it is hard for them to take in information. As one woman said, 'When I was first diagnosed, I'd say, "I'm not like the rest of them, I'm not schizophrenic, I'm not like that." But when you're sick with schizophrenia, you don't process the information.' Nevertheless, participants feel that it would have been helpful to have been told, for example, that what they were experiencing were delusions. As one woman said, 'Nobody, *nobody* was telling me I was suffering from delusions. They had me thinking that I had developed a second personality, but I didn't. It was a delusion, it wasn't real. It was the *idea* that I had a second personality.' In spite of now having information about schizophrenia, one participant noted that, in some ways, he is still in denial. 'I still have a hard time dealing with the fact that, yes, I have this condition. I'm still in denial and I probably always will be, because who wants to be this way?'

Interaction with Medical Professionals

Many of the participants had very painful stories to tell about their interactions with medical professionals, both in outpatient care and in institutions, when they felt their concerns were not heard or addressed or when they were not treated with respect and dignity. Participants felt resentment towards their doctors because of what they feel is a lack of compassion. They want to be treated with respect, and that means that they want medical professionals not only to supply information, but also to listen to and respond to their concerns. One man described his frustration in communicating his concerns to his doctors: 'My doctors are making me feel like it's a brick wall, and I want to strangle my doctor but I can't, it's against the law…. And until I change doctors I guess I feel like a guinea pig and like I'm hitting brick walls. It's very frustrating and I'm tired of feeling that way. I just want to be heard, I guess, about the subject.' One person described her view that some doctors adopt a superior stance and are not willing to take time to answer questions – 'They think they're gods and that what they say is gospel.' Another told a story about his new psychiatrist cleaning his nails during their appointments rather than attending to what he was saying. Another said, 'It seems like psychiatrists, their main thing is, is your brain okay and are you functioning mentally. Then after that they don't really care about side effects, physically what's happening, or anything else. You're not really treated as a whole person.' One participant asked to be heard by all her medical practitioners, saying, 'I want them to listen a hell of a lot better than they do.'

Most of the participants had been hospitalized at one time or another in various kinds of psychiatric institutions. While some of them found their time there helpful, others had some of their worst experiences. They told many stories about how they were ignored, treated harshly, looked down upon, and sometimes regarded as 'less than human.' They also talked about how they were made to feel like criminals when they were hospitalized, treated as though it was their fault that they were sick. As one participant put it,

> I felt criminalized in the [hospital]. They took away my clothes and my privileges. You get treated like a criminal. But it's not my fault. It's the illness. They gave me a shot and put me in a side room when I thought they were the Mafia. They were very rough. It really hurt. I told the psychiatrist, but he got mad and yelled at me. They left me overnight, with no mattress, just a pillow and a blanket. They don't care how much torture it is.

They were also often ignored by the very doctors and nurses who were supposed to help them. Here is what one participant said:

> You go up to the nurses' desk and they all ignore you. They don't talk to you, they put their heads down and continue to do whatever. They don't

even look at you or acknowledge you. It's like you're the invisible man on that soap commercial. And that's how they treat you. We're human. They think we don't hear, they think we don't process, but we're aware when we're being treated inhumanely.

Positive Experiences with Medical Professionals

The participants described much more positive treatment experiences when their medical professionals made an effort to develop open and empathic relationships that moved in the direction of Fisher's ideal. Communication in both the informational and the relational senses is central to these experiences and brings our four themes of diagnosis, medication, support, and interaction together in the lives of people diagnosed with schizophrenia. When people receive a definitive diagnosis, get information about medications and available support, and are treated with dignity and respect, they begin to feel much more accepting of their situation. They start to understand the need to take their medications and to look after themselves, and they start to see ways to deal with their situation.

Many participants described doctors who have helped them to get well and stay that way, and many are currently seeing doctors with whom they feel they have a good rapport. As one person said, 'My doctor knows how I'm feeling. He knows that I sometimes have my down days and my up days.' Their doctors, unlike ones they may have had in the past, listen to their problems and respond to them. Some of the participants referred to their doctors and other mental health professionals as their friends, 'professional' friends who help them accept and cope with having schizophrenia. They appreciate being involved with people who will listen to their concerns and genuinely attempt to respond to them. One woman, who was hospitalized during the time the research was taking place, returned to the group and described how different this experience was from her previous hospitalizations: 'My experience this time when I was in the hospital was really different. My doctor was doing something with my medications and I was really upset. So he explained it all to me. I said, "I understand why you made the change." And he said "Thank you for understanding."'

Some of the participants recognize that it is important not only for their doctors to develop a good relationship with them, but also for them to be open to what their doctors have to say. As one man said, 'You've got to have the right attitude, though, when you're talking to [medical people]. Because they have feelings too, just like anybody else, and they want to see the person that they're talking to is understanding them.' Many also feel that they must contribute to their own treatment. One person, looking back over his treatment, says that having his diagnosis disclosed to him by his doctors and getting information to help him understand the illness was important in becoming mentally well, but just as important was admitting to himself that he had schizophrenia and assuming responsibility for looking after himself. Another spoke about how he believed that his doctors could only help him if he was willing to help himself:

> The psychiatrist is only as good as your own improvement ... I feel I have to make a contribution, I have to work on my problems. [My doctor] allowed me to have my problems, to solve my problems. He helped to enhance my quality of life as a result. He made the good things better and he helped me to understand the bad things.

Another person also talked about her responsibility to participate in her treatment, saying that she feels the most important thing she has learned is that it is her responsibility to know about her illness and to take control of her own treatment. However, she points out that this can only happen if medical professionals are willing to listen: 'We [doctors and patients] need to have a working relationship where we both are respected for our opinions ... Before it was just one-way communication, now it's starting to be two-way.' Participants acknowledged that, with the help of their medical professionals and support systems, they have done better than many people diagnosed with schizophrenia in keeping themselves well and off the streets. As one participant noted, 'You know, everyone sitting here is a success story, 'cause for every one of us here, there's many, many people that are not doing well. We have the best life and everything available for us. We should count our blessings.'

Discussion

If there is one clear message that emerges from the research it is that communication with medical professionals, in both the informational and relational senses, is pivotal in the lives of people diagnosed with schizophrenia. Participants' early experiences with medical professionals include feelings of confusion and frustration produced by conflicting diagnoses, inadequate explanations of medications and their side effects, lack of information about schizophrenia, and inadequate support. Getting information about diagnosis, medication, and available support helps people diagnosed with schizophrenia to feel more positive about their experiences with medical professionals. It also is essential in coming to terms with having and learning to live with schizophrenia. The feelings of participants about their experiences with medical professionals are also closely tied to the quality of their interactions, both in and out of institutions, especially whether or not their concerns are heard and addressed. People diagnosed with schizophrenia want to be regarded by medical professionals as human beings deserving of the same dignity and respect as people with other kinds of illness. They want to be partners in decision-making about their own medical treatment. They are well aware that their behaviour while ill may make it difficult for medical professionals (and anyone else, for that matter) to regard them sympathetically and that being cooperative and having a 'good attitude' makes it more likely that they will get good treatment from medical professionals. But as one group member pointed out, it is hard to have a good attitude when you are ill, and medical professionals' memories of their behaviour while ill can lead to their being treated without respect even after they start to get better.

The burden of establishing good relationships must lie with medical professionals. When people are diagnosed with schizophrenia, they not only have no idea what is wrong with them, they are also unable to manage their interactions with others. People diagnosed with schizophrenia should not have to advocate for humane and respectful interaction. If a good relationship is to develop, it requires a concerted effort by professionals to work towards Fisher's mutual, educative exchange in their relationships with people diagnosed with schizophrenia. The kind of interaction that the research group members are asking for, in fact, requires service providers to turn over some of the control of the therapeutic process to people diagnosed with schizophrenia. As our results show, people diagnosed with schizophrenia are most likely to feel they are having a good experience with their medical professionals when they receive recognition that their perspective has a legitimate place in the practitioner-patient relationship, when they receive acknowledgment of their right to choice and self-determination in their treatments, and when they feel that they are included as respected partners in their treatment rather than regarded as passive recipients of treatment. This is not the traditional approach to the treatment of schizophrenia, but it is essential. The lives of people diagnosed with schizophrenia depend on it.

Here are the recommendations the research group members formulated for how they would like to be treated by medical professionals.

Recommendations for Medical Professionals

- It is your responsibility as medical professionals to communicate well with us. We have schizophrenia. We are mentally ill and we can't always manage our interactions with other people. You must teach us how to communicate well with you.
- Treat us with dignity and respect. No matter how sick and unstable we are, we are human beings. We are not a page out of the DSM (Diagnostic and Statistical Manual of Mental Disorders). We should not have to have an advocate to be treated like human beings. We deserve the respect, dignity, kindness, and normal treatment that other patients get.
- Tell us what is wrong with us. If someone has a heart attack or cancer, you tell them what is wrong with them, but with mental illness, you often won't tell us. We deserve the same kind of information as other ill people.
- When we come into hospital, don't take away our clothes and leave us naked in a tiny room. This humiliates us, and makes us feel degraded and criminalized.
- Let us rest when we are in hospital. We have had traumatic experiences and our bodies are adjusting to large doses of tranquillizing medications. You let other patients rest. We need the same kind of rest to get better.
- Don't send us out of town for treatment. This isolates us from our support network of family and friends and does not help us to get better. Find a way to treat us close to home.
- Listen to us and respond to our concerns about side effects and about how medications affect our physical health. Our physical health is as important as our mental health.
- Don't take power and control away from us. Empower us to be assertive and to make our own decisions. This will help us to adjust back into society. Give us the freedom to make our own choices.
- When you treat us, think about how it feels to have schizophrenia, and how it feels to take large doses of medications. Remember these words: *It's like walking in slavery.*

4 What We Learned: Housing for People Diagnosed with Schizophrenia (Results)

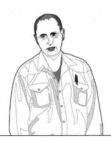

'Why do we have to struggle so hard to attain what should just be a normal right in society? We have a two-billion-dollar surplus in the province. Why can't we have affordable housing for everybody?' —Michele Misurelli

Stable housing is essential for people diagnosed with schizophrenia to be able to rebuild their lives. When people are worrying about where they will be sleeping next week or next month, or when they have to move every few weeks, they simply cannot develop independent and fulfilling lives. Achieving stability in housing requires many factors to come together in the lives of people diagnosed with schizophrenia. This constellation of factors includes financial supports, medication use, and treatment and family relationships. Most of the participants in our study experienced longer or shorter periods of being without a permanent home, but because of the difficulties of defining homelessness and capturing the variety of people's experiences, we have chosen not to use this word to describe their situations. Instead we use the terms *housing stability* and *instability* in our attempt to convey the complexity of people's housing experiences.

Most of the people in the research group and many of the people we interviewed live in some form of supported housing. This is housing provided by city and private agencies at subsidized or below-market rent, designated for people diagnosed with mental illnesses, either in apartment buildings or scattered in the community. Residents have access to a wide range of services to help them maintain their housing stability, including such things as a social worker on site from a few hours a week to twenty-four hours a day, organized social outings, and assistance with shopping and house-cleaning. In Calgary, the agencies that provide this housing require that people take their antipsychotic medication as prescribed, abstain from illegal drugs, and moderate their intake of alcohol. People who do not conform to these behavioural requirements are asked to leave the housing. That is, while the agencies offer much-needed assistance and care to people diagnosed with schizophrenia, they also exert a significant degree of control over the behaviour and lives of the people they serve.

Care and Control

Sociologist Nick Fox describes the paradoxical nature of care.[1] Care is almost always seen as a good thing, and the word carries almost no negative meanings. Control, however, seems to be an inevitable consequence of the provision of care, even if not intended by carers.[2] On the one hand, the act of caring comes from concern and a desire to provide for the needs of others. On the other hand, the disciplinary knowledge of the carer – that is, expertise in the field of mental health and knowledge of theories of care and professional practice – supplies 'the basis for the authority and power of those who practice care.'[3] Fox captures the control aspects of care in his description of what he calls the vigil of care in which the cared-for are continually subjected to 'the vigilant scrutiny of carers.'[4] For Fox, the vigil is more about power, surveillance, and control grounded in the professional knowledge of care givers than it is about the positive values typically associated with care. Fox also notes that an expectation of reciprocity underpins the provision of care: people who receive care must return something to the carer. People who receive care can manage this expectation by 'compliance or docility...or by "gratefulness" for the expertise of the carer.'[5] In order to receive housing services and medical treatment, people must agree to subject themselves to the surveillance and control that accompanies care, and they must express gratitude for that care. In short, they must be compliant.

Our research group used the Möbius strip (see figure 2) as a visual aid to represent for ourselves the relationship between care and control. A Möbius strip is a one-sided surface, made by taking a long strip of paper, giving it a half twist, and taping the ends together. To demonstrate that it has only one side, put a pencil anywhere on the strip, and, without taking the pencil off the paper, draw a line along the length of the strip. Soon you will find your pencil is on the opposite side of the paper

Figure 2. Möbius Strip: A Metaphor for the Relationship between Care and Control

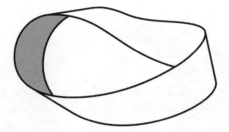

from the point at which you started. Keep drawing, still without taking the pencil off the paper, and you will find yourself back at the point you started. When you move your pencil along the strip, you see that the two sides blend into one, just as care blends effortlessly and inevitably into control. They are one and the same, although it at first seems that control is on the opposite side of the paper from care.

Dilemmas

This tension between care and control produces a complex set of dilemmas that people diagnosed with schizophrenia must negotiate in order to achieve stability. Members of the research group identified these dilemmas as the main theme arising from this set of interviews. Here is how they describe them:

- We are told that we are responsible for own recovery and for making our own choices. But we are limited by what service providers think are appropriate choices. The message we get is, 'Take responsibility, but do it our way.'
- We want to live normal lives, but in order to get services we must present ourselves as troubled in various ways. We must accept the label, *person with schizophrenia,* and the identity that goes with it in order to get the care we need and want. But once we have the label, we cannot get out from under it in any sphere of our lives.
- We must always accept and express gratitude for the help we receive, even when things are not really as we would like them to be. We are afraid of asking for even small changes for fear that we will lose what we have.

Figure 3. Housing Stability: Dilemmas of Care and Control

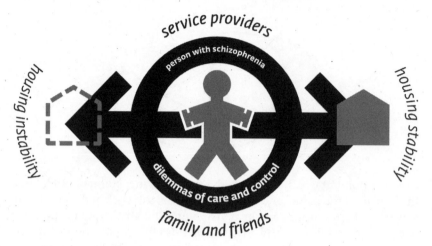

- We are reluctant to ask for help if we start to slip in our stability because we are afraid of losing our hard-won independence to the control of parents or 'the system.'

However, they are also deeply ambivalent about the control aspects of care. They resent the requirement that they be compliant but they sometimes also appreciate the control that accompanies care and they see benefits to themselves in having been forced into certain actions, such as taking medication.

Results

Our results show a complex dynamic pattern of housing stability and instability in which interactions with family members, roommates, individual service providers, and 'the system' are key factors in whether or not people diagnosed with schizophrenia achieve housing stability. We have tried to represent this complex pattern of interaction in figure 3.

The person with schizophrenia is in the centre of the diagram. People come into contact with the medical system, perhaps through hospitalization, are diagnosed with schizophrenia, and typically are prescribed antipsychotic medications. They may have already experienced conflict with family, friends, or roommates that has moved them in the direction of housing instability. They may also experience help and support from family members that moves them towards housing stability. They continue to be in contact with the medical system, and they also come into contact with housing service providers. At some times, people will have interactions with service providers that will help them to achieve housing stability. They will be willing to take on an identity as a person with schizophrenia and take medications, they will be willing and able to accept the control and surveillance inherent in care, they will have relationships with individual service providers that help them, and they will be able to accept the housing they are offered. At other times, they will receive housing services, but stay in situations of housing instability. They may not be willing to take on an illness identity and continue to take their medication, they may not get along with roommates they are assigned to, and they may not be able or willing to follow the rules of housing that is provided. For example, they may be unwilling to give up their pets or to abstain from illegal drugs.

As one group member put it, housing stability can change to instability in a flash. People can be asked to leave for various infractions such as not keeping the place clean or not attending twelve-step programs (e.g., Alcoholics Anonymous); they may encounter financial problems or may experience an increase in symptoms leading to inability to cope with housing rules; landlords or other people in the building may make life difficult for them so they leave the housing. Even doing well can lead to instability – people who are doing well can be asked to leave supported housing for housing in the community. Once people achieve long-term housing stability, and some consistent or at least manageable degree of wellness, they may begin to achieve more independence and become integrated into the community. They are able to volunteer, work, and may even leave the illness identity behind. But they may continue to experience the tension between care and control that characterizes their relations with the people and agencies that provide them with care.

Family Relationships

Many of the people diagnosed with schizophrenia interviewed for our study experienced a fairly long period in late adolescence and early adulthood characterized by housing instability: they had conflict with family members and left home during their teens, they had roommates who asked them to leave, they moved frequently, and they experienced periods of homelessness during which they stayed with friends (also known as couch surfing), lived in cars, roamed from town to town, lived in cockroach-infested slums, or stayed in shelters. Some moved as many as thirty times over the years. For some, long-term hospitalization for schizophrenia threatened their housing. Some described abusive relationships with parents and other family members that resulted in their leaving home. One woman described her youth this way: 'My family called me names, they'd lock me up in the closet. My dad doesn't even talk to me. He says "I want nothing to do with that girl, she's not my daughter. I disown her."' She ran away to Vancouver, where she found herself without money or housing, eventually hooking up with a pimp who provided housing in exchange for the sale of her sexual services. One man started using illegal drugs in his teens, which led to arguments with his mother and resulted in his leaving home before he was seventeen. One woman described conflict with her husband, who finally had her committed, put her belongings into storage, and disappeared from her life, leaving her with no place to go home to after release from hospital.

Others had conflict with roommates, which led to housing instability. One person told us, 'I'd have visual hallucinations and I would just go into my room and turn off the lights and lie down to calm myself down. But my roommate used to come in and she'd flip on the light and she'd grab me and she'd physically pull me up out of bed. She used to scream and yell at me, and say things to me like, "It's no wonder you have no friends."' Another objected to her roommate's drug use, was asked to leave, and was not able to find another affordable place. Another described having given his rent money to his roommates, who used it for drugs rather than giving it to the landlord, which resulted in his eviction. Another told of having given money for rent and food to a roommate who then put all his belongings outside and changed the locks, leaving him with no money and no place to go.

Many participants in our study also described supportive relationships with family or friends that have helped them to maintain stability in their lives. As one man said, 'Without parental units that care, I would have been homeless many, many times.' Another described the help she had received from her sister: 'She taught me how to look after money, she taught me how to do the house-cleaning and how to look after myself properly, and she helped me get my own place.' Another described a time when she was on the verge of losing her housing because she ran out of money: 'I couldn't pay my rent and I was very delusional. So my brother talked to my landlord and found out that I was about to be thrown out onto the street. He and the rest of my brothers and sisters went over to my place and packed up all my things and kept them at their places until I was able to move into a place in [another city].' Another got 'great references' from a former roommate, and so was able to find housing. Another described a boyfriend who said, 'You know, you just can't live like this.' He took her to the AISH office and helped her with the forms. She was then able to afford a small apartment.

However, even help and support from family can be seen as controlling and disempowering. One woman told us that after her mother died, her brother helped her out financially. But she said that he was never willing to discuss the financial arrangements with her: 'I don't know exactly to this day what he has worked out, but he helps me pay for the mortgage and I pay for the condo fees. But I don't exactly understand what it is and I often ask him. He just says "Don't worry about it," and he won't explain it to me.' Another woman tried to complain to her generally supportive family that her apartment manager entered her apartment without her permission. She recounted, 'They just said "It's your paranoia." When you have schizophrenia they can blame it on the paranoia and you can't fight back. It's not fair.' As one man said, 'Family likes to believe that you're doing well. It makes them feel good, so they're not open to listening.'

Getting into 'the System'

Coming into contact with the medical and housing provision systems means learning about a whole new world, rather like moving to a new and strange country. Many people have struggled with getting to know 'the system' and how they can fit into it. As one man said, 'In ten years as a mental health consumer, what I've learned is you flounder at first and it's almost worse. It's almost like an additional disease, just trying to understand all the agencies and what they want from you and what you're supposed to do and what your diagnosis is. And there's no one to kind of guide you through it all.' One of the primary things people have to learn is how to be 'compliant.' One man summed it up like this: 'You really have to submit to the system in order to receive benefit from it. If you do not want to submit to the system, then tough nuggies, good luck. Because you've got to play ball or you're not in the game.'

But many participants were genuinely grateful and pleased to have achieved a cooperative relationship with their service providers. For example, several people said that learning to trust their service providers was an issue for them. One man described his experience: 'I began to trust the guys and things started to work out from that point on. There was enough follow-through care after that with therapists and nurses. Part of it was that I started getting better, but starting to trust in the medical community, which I hadn't before, was a big part of it too.' Another man said, 'I found that as long as I told my worker the truth then there was a level of trust between me and the person working with me in the mental health system.' He also said he received praise from agency representatives for his willingness to comply with agency expectations. '"At least you tried to stay sober and at least you're taking your medication, at least you're doing something during the day." So I've found in my experience with the people in the mental health field, I've been getting credit for trying to help myself.' Learning how to cooperate with service providers was seen by these people as positive in helping them to move towards housing stability.

Medication

Most of our participants have come to appreciate the benefits of taking medication regularly. Many describe years of being on and off medications and connect this directly to their housing instability. One woman noted a reciprocal relationship between housing and medication: 'The funny thing is, stability in housing contributes to me being well too. It was kind of a circle that helped me…it kind of feeds each other, if I know my medication is stable and my housing is stable.' Because they see taking medication as a factor in maintaining stability and housing, many appreciate the control that is exerted to ensure that they comply with medication orders. They submit willingly to this control. As one said, 'When I'm off the medication, I get pretty sick. I need my medication because I get delusional. I have out-of-body experiences, I hear voices, I have episodes. I've got to be on my medication because it makes a load of difference.' She described her relationship with the Assertive Community Treatment team who come daily to her home to ensure she takes her medication and who have helped her 'maintain a stabilized state of mind.' This team also paid the deposit for the housing she is currently in and helped her move in. Another woman said that her greatest fear is that she will go off her medication, because she knows this would lead to hospitalization and possibly losing her home: 'It's a downhill slide, it's a shame. I don't want to shame my skin no more. I've had enough of it to realize that it's not fun. It seems fun at the time while you're off medication, but when you look back at it, you don't think so.' One man described his journey towards regular use of medication: 'Twenty years ago maybe you had a tenth, a fifth of the medications that you have now. The medications I was on, I was more or less blank. I didn't have the cognitive capacity to make good choices. So with medications that have worked over the last ten or fifteen years, I find housing and getting along in the system has improved a lot.'

One woman described what happened when she went off her medications a few years ago: 'They threatened that I'd have to leave [my housing] if I didn't comply. So I handed in my key and I left. Then the police came and they got on the bus and hauled me off the bus. It was kind of embarrassing that the police were involved.' She was taken to hospital and put back on her medication, which she now takes regularly. In some cases, people provide this kind of control for each other. One person described a living situation in which the other people in the building, all of whom have also been diagnosed with mental illnesses, provide the surveillance. When one resident went off his medications, the other residents got together to discuss his situation and began talking of trying to force him out of the building if he did not go back on his medications.

Financial Stability

Most of the people interviewed for our study are on AISH, the disability pension in Alberta. They are extremely grateful for the financial stability it provides, and there can be no doubt that this is an essential aspect of housing stability. As one woman said, 'If you can't pay your rent, you can't keep your house, and if you're sick, you can't keep your job. That's the way it works for me.' Getting onto AISH was a key turning point for many of our participants in achieving stability.

One man described his life as 'a bit tough' before AISH. He described being on Medical Welfare, which pays considerably less than AISH, as 'a bit difficult, because I couldn't smoke or do the things I wanted to, so I ended up picking butts off the street.' Another said that before being on AISH, 'Stability was a concern. If I had one week without income I had stress, and without loved ones, when you're in crisis it's huge, it's not minor, it's a crisis with a capital C. For those who have no loved ones, who have burnt bridges and feel that the very act of reaching out is too much, why not just slip between the cracks and pick bottles for a few years?' Another said, 'It was a big breakthrough when I was on AISH because I was always struggling for money.' Another told us how she planned for possible homelessness before AISH: 'I even had my boyfriend teach me how to live if I ever ended up homeless. He would take me to the bins behind houses. There's a lot of great things in the garbage, in the bins. We'd wear gloves and have coat hangers or sticks that you would use to pull things out. And the things you take out would only be really, really clean stuff. And then at the back of Safeway before they got the burner things in, you could get pretty good food too.'

It is clear that AISH has made a tremendous difference in the lives of the people we talked to. But it also provides another example of the control that accompanies care. Many of our interviewees expressed frustration with the surveillance they must submit to. To continue to receive AISH, recipients must submit their tax forms every year, report any additional income, and be available for random financial and personal audits in their own homes. People fear and resent the power that AISH workers have to cut them off and chafe under the control imposed on them. As one woman said, 'I find that they want to scrutinize my past in order for me to receive what I'm entitled to…. They hand you a page of personal questions and it's like, I just want stability, why are you sniffing my butt so much? You really start to feel less than human.' Another said, 'You can scrutinize me and I'll try to stand up to it, but you don't have to scrutinize my brother or my sister and my mother and the guy I was married to fifteen years ago.'

One man said that he had to attend appointments with Alberta Mental Health to continue to receive AISH. He said that his Alberta Mental Health worker told him, '"As long as you're working with us you're going to be okay. You can have your financial income as long as you work with us." That's part of the ground rules to be on AISH – I have to work with a Mental Health worker.' One woman described herself as being 'extra-nice' to her AISH worker, who has a reputation of being hard to get along with. As a result, she said, 'I haven't received any of the threatening letters' that others receive from AISH. This woman also complained about AISH procedures for clawing back benefits when she receives income from other sources, saying that this produces instability in her life and makes her reluctant to seek more employment. If she makes and reports money one month, it is taken out of her cheque the next month. If she doesn't make as much money in that next month, she then has to manage on less for that month. Another described her difficulty getting onto AISH: 'I was going to the library, doing research, and I ran into a booklet about welfare. It said, "To qualify for AISH you must have exhausted all resources within the community." I think now that I look back, that's why I was jumping through all the different hoops. They didn't put me on AISH until four years after my first [psychotic] break.'

Getting onto AISH was essential, but learning to manage the money also was important. One man described the challenges: 'I found that I would go out on spending sprees and spend until I had no money left in my account, and then I realized I didn't have any money for the rent. And that's when I started budgeting. I could do it one month but I couldn't do it the next month.' Here again we can see the ambivalence our participants feel about the control aspects of care. Several talked about the importance to their stability of the trusteeship relationship, in which individuals are required to turn over control of their finances to someone else. For example, one person said, 'I think we set up a dual account. I couldn't take money out unless I had the other person's signature. So I couldn't drink and do stuff like that. I felt that it was a good decision and a good choice that I made because I was not capable of seeing the consequences of my actions. I didn't see that I could end up, well, I guess I sort of did see that if I kept it up I would end up homeless.' Another described his situation: 'I get money on the weekend, so if I foul up, it's just for a week instead of a whole month.' Another man described how his ex-wife acts as his trustee and manages his money for him, even though she is now living with another man. These people have accepted and even welcomed the control that ensures their financial stability. But as one woman said, 'I'm grateful for the help, but I am frustrated that I can't manage my money myself.'

Relationships with Housing Agencies

Relationships with housing agencies also illustrate the dilemmas of care and control. A number of participants identified a particular person at an agency as being the most important factor in helping them find stable housing. One woman happened into the Alberta Alcohol and Drug Abuse Commission office, where a counsellor suggested to her, 'You know, there is another life besides this life.' This counsellor was instrumental in 'helping me to make a decision that I didn't want to live this kind of life anymore. I finally said no for the very first time. I never said no but this time I did.' One person was driven around by his AISH worker to find a new apartment. Another was recommended by an agency representative to a supported housing complex that he still lives in. One told us that AISH threatened to cut her off while she was in hospital for a long period, which threatened her housing. Her psychiatrist talked to her AISH worker and resolved the problem. Another said that her psychiatrist had advocated for her with a housing agency. These service providers were remembered as instrumental in helping people to achieve housing stability.

On the other hand, some aspects of the relationship between agency service providers and our participants were seen as ineffective or controlling, leading to conflict with service providers. One man said that, in his experience, 'most agencies are ineffective in connecting you or empowering you in your search for housing. They'll say, "Well, look in the paper, or sucks to be you, good luck." Proactive is not in the language of many agencies. They'll refer you, but will they champion your purpose or your cause or will they stand beside you? No, they'll just point you in the right direction and say, "Happy Trails."' A number of our participants described situations in which treatment or services were withheld when the person did not behave in ways that the service provider thought appropriate. A number of participants told of having been kicked out of programs or shelters because of their behaviour. For example, one man said he had been kicked out of a shelter for getting into a fight with another man. Another told of being kicked out of two treatment programs for 'acting odd.' Another said that a particular program did not want to let him back in because of his drug use. This same man said that he had been told that he 'was completely defiant' about the plans that the agency had set up for him. He wanted to change his financial arrangements (the agency was acting as his trustee) so that his mother would be his trustee. The agency told him that they wanted nothing more to do with him. 'If that's the way he feels, then he's cut off.' Another woman was threatened with losing her housing if she did not keep the place clean. She was upset because she knew that others in her building had received help to clean their places, but she did not seem to be eligible for that help.

One woman, who has diabetes as well as schizophrenia, told us about how she had waited three years to get into subsidized housing. But because she was not taking her insulin as prescribed by her doctor, he insisted that she move out of her subsidized apartment and into a group home where her insulin regimen could be monitored. However, she could not take her daughter with her to a group home and so went to live with a family acquaintance who soon asked her to leave. This was the beginning of a period of housing instability during which she moved thirty times and lived in substandard places, one of which had mould, mice, and mushrooms growing through the carpet. She now says, 'Listening to my doctor was the biggest mistake I ever made.'

Other people felt they could not accept the housing they were offered. For example, agencies that provide supported housing typically do not permit pets, so people who are not willing to give up their pets cannot be accommodated in supported housing. As one woman said about her cat, 'She's my whole world, I just can't give her up. I live for her. So because I had a cat I had to go into slum housing. ' People described being placed with roommates not of their own choosing, which sometimes did not work out. One man described his experience in a group living situation: 'I lived in an approved home for a couple of years, but I block that out of my mind because it was such a horrible experience. You start off by being agreeable and then you find yourself becoming compliant. It's done through a bunch of rules and social policies that are the vehicle for developing submission and a lack of self-worth. That's probably the one thing that really worries me, is the idea of ever ending up in one of those places again.'

Many of our participants told us about situations in which they had problems with the landlord or housing manager. Several told us of managers who entered their apartments without permission. One person recounted, 'The managers would come in anytime they wanted to and it scared me. They just came in and they stole my toilet paper, they stole my sheets, they stole my towels.' Another person could never get his fridge fixed, no matter how many times he asked. He said, 'Once you stand up and speak your mind and say you have no right to do this, they turn around and they berate you, put you down, call you names. So that's why I'm afraid to say something because then I'll get on their bad side. If I get on their bad side my place won't be painted.' They also complained about agency rules that prevented people from getting the help they felt they needed. For example, one woman told us that 'The ILS workers [social workers in her supported housing building] don't have much power. They can't take you and drive you to the hospital if they think you're not doing well. They have to go through all the bureaucratic rigamarole.'

Sometimes even doing well can lead to instability. Agencies may decide that people no longer need the support provided by their housing settings. One told us, 'My psychiatric nurse along with three or four workers came and did some kind of progress report and they decided that it was time for me to move on.' A member of the research group says she does not want to ask anyone about whether a person can become too high-functioning for her supported apartment building for fear that someone might find out how well she is doing and ask her to leave. 'They don't really support in some ways the idea of being very high-functioning. I don't even like the word high-functioning.' Referring to the arrows in our diagram, she said, 'As long as you're in those arrows you're not in control, your supports are in control. Not until you become independent in your own housing can you move away and beyond those arrows. But even then you still have to live in fear of them.'

Achieving Stability

When individuals successfully navigate the rocky shoals of care and control and achieve a degree of permanence in their housing, they are free to develop other aspects of their lives and integrate into the wider community. One woman said that now that she could count on stable housing, she had started to volunteer and participate in community activities. She said that many of the other people in her building (who have also been diagnosed with mental illnesses) have had the same experience. Another woman started teaching an evening craft course for a continuing education program, where her identity as a person with schizophrenia is not relevant. Some are taking university courses offered by a street-front program at a city shelter and are working towards university transfer. But even these achievements are bittersweet. As one man said, 'I remember when I was younger, in my late teens, early twenties, before my illness grabbed hold of me, I was concerned about how to fit into this society, how to fit into the system. Now thirty years later with the help of Alberta Mental Health, I've found that I'm really in the middle of the system that I wanted to get into in the first place, except as a recipient instead of as a contributor.'

Discussion

As our results show, the paradoxical nature of care produces dilemmas for people diagnosed with schizophrenia that underlie all their interactions with service providers. It is easy for service providers to see recipients of medical and housing services as simply 'noncompliant' when they do not behave 'appropriately' and to think that they do not want or deserve help or services. We suggest that they can instead be seen as struggling to negotiate the complex dilemmas that being cared for presents and to reconcile the deep ambivalence they feel about the control aspects of care. If people reject care because of the surveillance and control they would have to submit to, this is not simply noncompliance. It may even be a reasonable response to circumstances that people without a diagnosis of schizophrenia would not be willing to tolerate. Achieving housing stability depends as much on the service provider and the care provided as it does on the recipient. Failure to achieve housing stability is not just the 'fault' of individuals who need to shape up and take some responsibility for their situations. Agencies must also take some responsibility for polices that produce people as problems through the imposition of behavioural and other rules and deprive them of housing when they do not follow the rules.

The dilemmas of care are not likely to disappear – it would be quite unrealistic to think that a long history of care as vigil can be erased. However, Fox offers the possibility that care can be different. He points out that 'the vigil's disciplinary power is not situated outside the care setting – in policy or institutions ... – but in the everyday practices of care, in the contact between the carer and the cared-for.'[6] That is, the character of care and the outcome in the lives of people receiving care can be found in the interaction between the care giver and the care receiver and in the way care is experienced and responded to by both the individual provider and the recipient. Fox describes care in the form of what he calls a gift, in which generosity is substituted for the vigil. Care as gift is freely given without expectation of reciprocity in the form of docility or gratitude, a gift that allows people to achieve personal growth and actualization. 'This gift enables and empowers, it allows the recipient of the gift to "become other," to establish a new subjectivity.'[7] Fox acknowledges the difficulty of putting care-as-gift into practice, particularly as he cannot provide a formula for doing so. In fact, providing such a formula might run the risk of returning care to the realm of vigil.

The onus to change the circumstances of care and to make it a gift is on medical and housing service providers rather than on service recipients diagnosed with schizophrenia. And it is in fact through Fisher's uncoerced, mutual, educative communication that care can become a gift that will enable people to take up the responsibility for their own lives and to find meaning and purpose in their activities. Communication, in both the informational and relational senses, entails all of those things that the research group members ask for in their recommendations in our first project: receiving information about what is happening to them; not being treated in degrading and dehumanizing ways; having their concerns heard and attended to; being included in treatment decisions; not being asked for or forced into unthinking compliance; being enabled to make their own choices; and being regarded as people who can accomplish something in life. Communication based on recognition of their essential humanity and their right to be treated as individuals deserving of respect and dignity is the essence of the gift and brings us full circle in our research. Care, control, and communication are intertwined in the lives of people diagnosed with schizophrenia and shape their everyday experiences in the medical and housing systems. The gift of care through communication offers a way to make people diagnosed with schizophrenia equal partners in decision-making about their own lives. It helps them to rebuild independent and fulfilling lives and find a way out of the dependence/independence paradox.

Recommendations for Housing Providers

Group members formulated the following recommendations for housing service providers.

Providing Care

- Have a central agency for the city that knows about all the housing options for people diagnosed with mental illnesses. Make sure that one person from this agency follows someone right through the system, A to Z, from homeless to housed, so people do not get lost in the system.
- Provide an advocate to mediate disputes between people diagnosed with mental illnesses and housing providers or landlords.
- Provide more education about mental illness to housing service providers and landlords. Many lack compassion and do not treat us with respect and dignity.
- Provide education for families about different options and offer more support for families. Families can be an important stopgap that catches you before you fall to the streets.
- Provide support to help us as we get more independence. We are very fragile when we start to do things and need help with doing

taxes, saving money, learning about insurance, learning about nutrition, and providing for ourselves in the future.

Reducing Control While Providing Care

- Don't ask us for compliance. Work with us to help us make choices but do not tell us what we have to do. We do not want to be forced to live the way you think we should live.
- Don't make us share with roommates unless we are willing to.
- Don't ask us to expose our whole lives. The fact that we are living with a mental illness on a disability pension does not mean that you have a right to intrude into our lives.
- Simplify the AISH system. Right now, if you start to work, the paperwork required by AISH is overwhelming. It makes you not want to work. As you start working, it should be easier instead of more complicated.

Expanding Access to Housing

- We should be able to live where we want to live. Most of us dream of living in our own homes in the community. Help us to make this a reality.
- Do not move us without our consent. Housing should be permanent. We should not have to move just because we reach age sixty-five or don't 'fit in' to particular housing.
- Provide more different ways of housing people, including people who have pets. Housing should be flexible to accommodate people's needs.
- We need more affordable housing and society has to make this a priority. Provincial and federal governments could give tax incentives for affordable housing or require that builders make a certain percentage of their units affordable housing. We must find the political will to have more affordable housing.

5 Our Photovoice Project Searching for Sanctuary: What Home Means to Me

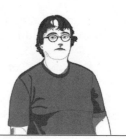

WITH MONIQUE SOLOMON

'I think that capturing phenomena in photographs, graphically, is as powerful as words. When you depict it, it goes hand-in-hand with the written word, it adds to the flavour, the theme.' —Jamal Ali

'In Street Talk (Calgary's street newspaper),[1] I saw some pictures that were taken and one just hit me. It was a cupboard. It was all empty and the only thing in it was a jar of peanut butter that had just a little bit of peanut butter in it. It had scrapes in the peanut butter jar and that really hit me that they were trying to make that last for another week.' —Laurie Arney

This chapter tells the story of our photography project, which took place during the time that we were working on the housing project. This project illustrates yet another way for people diagnosed with schizophrenia to be involved in research. In our interviews and focus groups in the housing project, we asked our interviewees to talk about what home means to them. This became a question of great interest to the research group members and they decided to use photography to explore in more depth what home means to them. We used a method known as photovoice,[2] in which silenced or under-represented people photograph the realities and challenges of their lives in order to stimulate critical reflection, raise awareness, and promote social change. Our objective was to increase awareness about the importance of secure housing as an essential factor in maintaining wellness for people diagnosed with schizophrenia. Other photovoice studies on homelessness have focused on the harsh realities of life on the street or in homeless shelters. The members of our group wanted instead to explore what it means to have stable housing, from their vantage point as people who now have secure housing after having experienced housing instability. Through their photographs, discussion, and analysis, the members of the group show how the everyday aspects of home that most of us take for granted are integral to their ability to stay well.

The photographs in our project are simple – the front door of an apartment, a washer and dryer, a book-shelf filled with bric-a-brac, old family photos hanging on a beige living room wall. But the meanings attributed to them by the group members convey the value and importance of the places they call home. Many of the photos show private aspects of their lives, illustrating that being involved in a photography project such as this requires participants to reveal things that might make them vulnerable in some way. Paradoxically, however, opening themselves up also reduces their vulnerability, first by enabling them to articulate for themselves the importance of home in maintaining wellness in their own lives, and then by increasing their confidence in their ability and right to present their views for a larger audience.

Photovoice

Photovoice was developed by public health researcher Carolyn Wang in the 1990s. She describes it as integrating health promotion principles, feminist theory, theoretical literature on education for critical consciousness, and non-traditional approaches to documentary photography.[3] As a method of critical expression, photovoice has three main goals: 'to enable people to record and reflect on their personal and community strengths and concerns; to promote critical dialogue and knowledge about personal issues through group discussions of photographs; and to reach policymakers.'[4] Initially, the method was proposed as an inclusive way to assess the health needs of women in developing countries and to aid in the development of effective and appropriate health promotion strategies.[5] Photovoice has been taken up by those seeking visual means for raising awareness about the personal, cultural, and socio-economic circumstances of marginalized groups.[6] The method has become popular at least in part because of its simplicity – almost anyone with a camera can take part.

Taking photographs is a straightforward way to produce research data that represents people's everyday lived experiences. But asking ordinary people to take and analyse photos stands outside the usual 'scientific' understanding of legitimate ways to gather data and challenges the stranglehold that the elite research community has maintained over how knowledge is produced and disseminated. Popular participation in knowledge production contests the exclusive right of expert researchers to determine how research problems are defined and studied, has the potential to alter who legitimately has the right to collect information and produce knowledge, and challenges the 'very definition of what constitutes knowledge.'[7] It asserts ordinary people as a legitimate and important source of expertise and allows people who have historically had little power to articulate their experiences and determine how they are represented. When research participants set the agenda, guide the direction of the research, and present their work on their own terms, they reframe social issues in light of their direct experience.

A number of photovoice studies of homelessness demonstrate the insights that this approach to research can produce. For example, researchers in London provided cameras to people who were homeless and followed up with in-depth interviews in order to produce visual and textual data about how people not only survive but make a life on city streets.[8] Wang and her colleagues used photovoice to enable men and women living in a homeless shelter in Ann Arbor, Michigan, to document their daily struggles.[9] In Calgary, Alberta, photovoice was used to explore the meaning of home to women living in a homeless shelter.[10] Photovoice has also been used as a way for service providers to engage young people experiencing poverty and homelessness.[11] These projects offer an understanding of homelessness from the perspectives of those who experience it and contribute to new ways of thinking about homelessness. Taking part in photovoice also has personal value for the photographers, enabling them to 'see' themselves, their lives, and their communities from new perspectives.

Getting Started

Our photovoice project took place over the course of four months, between January and April of 2006. Six members of the housing research group took part – Laurie, Jamal, Cindy, Michele, Claude, and Mary. Two additional people who had taken part in a focus group for the housing project joined us for the photovoice project. The group met twice a month for an hour before the meetings for the housing project. This schedule enabled group members to attend all research-related meetings on one day. The meetings took place in the late afternoon so there was an opportunity for the group to enjoy a meal together before the main research project meetings. This turned into an important link between meetings and gave the participants a chance to chat about the meeting topics in a relaxed atmosphere. Graduate assistant Monique Solomon planned the topics for each meeting, but the development of ideas and flow of conversation were guided by the interests of the group members. The meetings were recorded and transcribed so that excerpts from group discussions could be used in presentations of the project.

During the first meeting, we discussed the principles and goals of photovoice, and the group talked about why they were interested in taking photos. The focus of the meeting was to consider how our photovoice project could contribute to a new understanding of issues faced by people diagnosed with schizophrenia. Members of the group noted that their interviews for the larger project were a powerful way to explore issues, but it was difficult to hear so many distressing stories. The group embraced the idea of looking for positive things that signified the importance of a secure, stable home as a contributing factor in mental well-being. As Mary said, 'Before we did the photo project, we listened to some very, very real interviews and people were in really bad positions. I think that struck all of us, how lucky we were to have a home and maintain a home, and being able to do so now because we're mentally well enough or we have an income.'

To generate a discussion about the power of photographs, Monique showed some generic photographs that she had cut out of various magazines. Members of the group chose photographs that they liked and talked about why they liked them. They then brainstormed specific themes that could be presented in their own photographs including hope, transitions, and healing. Group members suggested they could take pictures of such things as running water, a bed, the lock on a door, food, and the Bible. They also considered potential audiences for the project, including housing and funding agencies, politicians, the media, and the general public. We laid out a timeline for the project of about four months.

During the second meeting, the group focused on the practical issues of taking photographs. They expressed concerns about the ethics of taking pictures of people not involved in the project, or of taking pictures of signs, for example in public places or in front of places where they had once lived. Ethics approval had been granted by the university for the project and the photographers had signed informed consent forms. To address the concerns raised by the group, we created a permission form for photographs of people or of private properties or signage. Group members also raised more personal issues. They were worried about the way their homes looked and about how sharing photographs of their homes might impact their funding status. For example, one person was concerned that someone might think she 'had too much' for a person on social assistance when they saw a picture of a colour TV that she had saved for months to buy. Despite these concerns, the group members wanted to continue with the project. The value of participatory action research is that the participants themselves are aware of and work collaboratively to address these practical and ethical issues.

We also talked about how to use the camera and how to take good photographs. In the week before this meeting, Monique had tested one of the small disposable cameras (35 mm, 27 exposure) we were using for the project. She brought in photos she had taken of various places on the university campus so we could talk about the camera's quirks and so the group could see the quality of the photographs it would take. She reviewed strategies for taking interesting photographs such as changing the angle of the camera or moving closer to or farther from a scene. Everyone received a handout of tips and instructions on using the camera and then went home to take their photos. Two weeks later, they returned to hand in their cameras, which were taken in for developing.

Analysing the Photographs

In photovoice projects, the photographers drive the analysis.[12] The photographs are the data and the analysis occurs as the photographers consider both the content of the photos and the experience of taking them. They select photographs they feel are most relevant or simply ones they like best, and individually and collectively consider which ones to display. Their choices and the meanings they attach to the photographs inform the analysis. They identify the main impressions and sentiments that the photographs convey and decide on the key social and community ideas represented in them. They also attend to the process of doing the research – what they value (or not) about the research experience and how this influences their decisions about how to present the photos.

Taking the Photographs

The members of the photovoice group agreed that the experience of taking photographs was not quite as straightforward as they had anticipated. Some had challenges with the camera flash or advancing the film. They weren't sure if the camera was really capturing the images they wanted. Interestingly, none of the photographers used the whole roll of film. The group agreed that it was difficult to 'know what exactly to take pictures of.' Others were concerned about the way their homes would look to others. As one person said, 'My home isn't the way I want it to be, but I took the pictures anyway.' Laurie's journal describes her experience of taking the photos:

> **Laurie's Journal, 19 January 2006.** *We went over how to use the camera and some of the themes we could use while photographing our homes. I had a great time when I got home. Spirituality is a big one for me. I photographed the golden angel my sister sent me for Christmas. Saying prayers can be very difficult for me at times because of the voices. With my golden angel I can put written prayers in her basket. Also I love my fairy and candle. I light it at night and have a cup of tea and relax. I had to take some pictures of my paintings. A big loss for me when I moved was losing my cat Whiskey. I am not allowed pets here so my daughter painted a picture of him for me. I had lots of fun taking pictures of my place, even my meds.*
>
> **Laurie's Journal, 2 February 2006.** *I went to the photovoice group. I was listening to others talk about their experience of photographing their homes. Their emotions were mixed. Seems pictures could trigger really positive experiences or ones of loss.*

Reviewing the Photographs

One of the highlights of the project occurred when the members of the group saw their photographs for the first time. Two sets of prints had been developed from each camera. Each photographer received a copy of their prints and a small album to store them in. The second set of prints was reviewed by the group as a whole. There was a sense of fellowship and excitement. Everyone talked about the photographs they had taken, remarking spontaneously about why they had taken certain photographs and what the images represented. They were eager to see what others had done and expressed enthusiasm for each others' photographs. Laurie describes the experience:

Laurie's Journal, 23 February 2006. The photographs we had taken of our homes were developed. This was a fun night. Everyone was excited to see how the pictures they had taken turned out. We all tried to pick out our favourite five photos. Then we shared why they were our favourites. It was great to see what others had chosen. Images that they had chosen had a lot of memories and emotion attached to them, from images of family photos, pets, favourite areas, to a child's computer. We learned a lot more about each other. I found myself very excited when it became my time to share. I realized my home means so much to me. I spend a lot of time alone in my apartment. So I surround myself with a lot of objects that remind me of people I love and have been kind to me. As an artist, it is the space I create in. I love to be surrounded by that which inspires me. I need to feel safe. Feeling safe is very important to me.

Here is some of what group members said about their photos. In these brief narratives, the group members provide context and background for a deeper consideration of the connections between home and well-being:

- *I took a picture of my kitchen because it's the heart of my home where I cook all my food, and it reminds me of being satisfied, having plenty, and not being in need.*
- *That's my number. I wanted to say, 'That's mine, apartment 402.'*
- *Because I can't have pets, I have a lot of plants. I get very attached to them.*
- *This is the view from my apartment. There's a park right across the street where we can take our dogs.*
- *The bed's important because I like my soft pillow and my cuddly blankets.*
- *Behind it you see my hobby, sewing. There's a great big pile of material.*
- *I've got the recycling box because I really believe in recycling.*
- *The couch is important when I want to watch TV.*
- *I took a picture of the thermostat because that's important in the winter.*
- *This is a picture of a beautiful tree outside my place. It's wonderful and a great big huge tree, so I go out on the balcony for its shade.*

Selecting the Photographs

At the next meeting, the photographers chose five favourites from their own collections of photos and briefly shared with the group why they liked them. Then all of the favourites were spread randomly on a table and everyone took a second look at the photographs. Each member of the group was encouraged to choose one or two favourites that were not their own. The group followed this process in order to narrow down the large number of photographs. This process left us with a manageable number of photographs and helped to guide a more focused analysis. Laurie describes this activity:

> *Laurie's Journal, 2 March 2006. Monique brought all our favourite photos together and then some. We picked our themes; then we chose the photographs that resonated with the themes. My first pick was the photo of Mary's cat. Having to give up my cat so that I could live in my apartment still bothers me. The cat represented choices, companionship, and nurturing. My apartment is great and I appreciate living here so much. Still it is important no matter where you live to have choice and control over your own environment. As we continued to choose photos around different themes, it was insightful seeing group members' choices, how different sometimes the images could be. I learned more about myself and what was important to me; this was shared with the group. I feel on common ground when I participate in this – it is a good feeling.*

After their initial selections were made, the group agreed that each member would choose one photograph to be used in a conference presentation later that year. However, when they saw the initial PowerPoint slides for the presentation showing just one photograph per person, they were dismayed that so few of their photos appeared in the presentation. We decided instead to create a collage using the favourite photographs from each member of the group. Short narratives accompanied the collages to contextualize the photographs for the audience. Group members were much happier with this. Laurie describes:

> *Laurie's Journal, 6 April 2006. Monique went through the photos we had picked and put them in a format that we could all view on screen. We all helped with giving a short biography touching on when our housing was unstable and how it impacted our lives, and the gratefulness of being in stable housing now. We talked about the different themes we are using in our project. We made different comments about the photographs and what they meant to us. Michele suggested we use more photographs. A lot of us liked that idea. We brainstormed a name for our project. It was hard to find the right words to express all that we had been doing and feeling in this group. The closest we came to agreeing on something for a title was 'Searching for Sanctuary – What Home Means to Me' or 'Searching for Sanctuary – A Place to Call Home.'*
> *Laurie's Journal, 20 April 2006. Monique brought in a close to finished version for the group to see. Lots of photos - the first five favourites that each member*

had chosen from their own pictures. Lots of text had been added and each person read theirs aloud. The text was great in relating the different experiences of the group, showing how important the simple things in life are that most people take for granted. For me it felt good when photographs I had taken were used in the project, like the angel that represented spirituality for me, and to know it was important for others in the group also. They had their own photographs that showed spirituality and faith. It made me realize it is very important to have your home, where you can surround yourself with your own beliefs that give you strength.

Discussing the Photographs

Through their photographs and discussions, the group members articulated what they value about home: sanctuary, privacy, safety and security, spirituality, and community. They also expressed their appreciation for their current circumstances. The sections that follow present comments group members made in our meetings as we discussed these various themes.

SANCTUARY

- *I think we found out home means about the same for all of us. It's a sanctuary and it's a nice place if you want to entertain or do whatever.*
- *I had a lot of nature scenes. I love nature. The serenity of it just keeps me at peace. I've lived in my house since October. It's just a nice place to live. It's well maintained and I don't have to do anything.*
- *I like being able to put my paintings up around my apartment and this shows a little bit of the paintings too. It's great being able to paint and put my artwork up.*
- *The kitchen is really important to me because lots happens in the kitchen. You cook or you visit. I had a small party at my place and we had lots of fun that night and that means a lot to me. I guess more than any other room in the house, the kitchen's my favourite.*
- *Being home is like a sanctuary.*

PRIVACY

Participants had to make choices about privacy. Their homes give them the ability to live their lives away from the eyes of others. But showing their photos means they reveal private aspects of their lives. This dilemma was highlighted in the decision one participant made about photos that her boyfriend (also a member of the group) had taken of her enjoying the luxury of a bubble bath in the privacy of her own home. Her boyfriend said that he 'made sure there was enough suds to cover all bases.' She said, 'At first I thought the photos were just funny, because I thought, you're at home, you can do what you want, you can have a bath.' After some reflection, she asked that the photos not be used in the poster version of the project because 'I thought somebody might misunderstand the pictures, so then I was concerned about that.' When Colin McDonald, our graphic designer, suggested that he could crop the picture so that only her head and a few bubbles showed, she thought that this was a good compromise between illustrating her privacy and maintaining it. This solution reduced her level of personal vulnerability and freed her to include the photographs on the poster.

SAFETY AND SECURITY

- *Safety and security was kind of the common thread. There were a lot of pictures of locks on the door. It just really makes you appreciative of what you have. I still think of the safety issue and how powerful a picture of a lock is. Everybody is entitled to have their privacy and shelter and a place where they can keep bad things out. That was one of the really powerful symbols to me.*
- *There was a time where I ended up in the hospital and all of my belongings were in storage and at that point I didn't know where I was going after I was released from the hospital. So, having my own apartment means wellness, the ability to take care of myself. And that means a lot for me; it's like a safety nest.*

SPIRITUALITY

- *There was so much in my home that it was hard to really single out what I wanted to take pictures of. I found that spirituality was really strong and I didn't realize that before, until I saw the photos. I realized that spirituality is something that we keep in our homes that we draw strength from. It's different for each of us, but it's really important to have a place where you can surround yourself in that way.*

COMMUNITY

- *I noticed Jamal had a lot of people in his pictures where I noticed I didn't have any people in mine. I was wondering, is that significant in some way? I find my house is more somewhere where I retreat to and then I go out and socialize from there, so I find that interesting. I'm inviting people in more but I found it interesting that I hadn't taken pictures of anyone. I found that I was questioning myself.*

- *Reflecting on the idea that some of us didn't have people (in the photos), it still conveys a sense of home because home is not the actual dwelling that you're living in, it's beyond, it's a community, the natural surroundings also. It's part of home, what you're in tune with, what makes you feel comfortable. So if there are pictures of scenery, a river and trees and you can see the mountains in the background, that's home to that person, a larger sense of home.*

THANKFULNESS

- *My life was chaos. I moved about twenty times in three years. I lived in a basement suite from hell. Now I have a brand new condo and I have peace, joy, and hope.*
- *I took a picture of my fridge because I know what it's like to be hungry. I'm thankful for the four hundred dollars I got, that I was able to fill my fridge and my meat freezer with food.* (Note: In 2005, every resident in Alberta received a $400 'bonus' from the government.)
- *I have a bed finally. I don't have to call it a bed from hell. I got a Sleep Country bed. I saved up for a few years to get this bed. But I got this bed and I have pretty good sleeps on this bed.*

Presenting the Photographs

The collages were presented by Laurie and Monique at a conference at York University in 2006. The final presentation for the project was a poster that included all 200+ photographs in miniature put together by Colin. Quotes from group members and from our interviews and focus groups about what home means appear beside the photos. The photo poster was framed and distributed to housing and mental health agencies in Calgary, providing a long-lasting opportunity for people to see our work. This poster has also been shown at numerous conferences and community events. Our work invites audiences to think about what home means and to draw their own connections between the photographs and the quotes about the meaning of home.

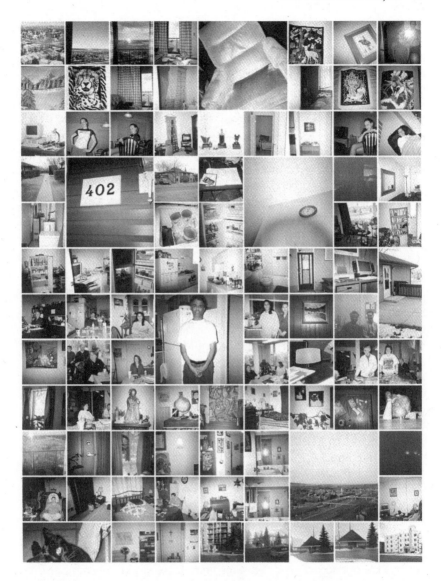

A section of the photovoice poster put together by Colin McDonald, created from photos taken by research group members.

Reflecting on the Photovoice Project

After we had completed the project, done our conference presentation, and distributed the poster to housing and mental health agencies in Calgary, the members of the group met again to discuss their experiences in the project. Several people commented on the way in which taking the photographs changed their perceptions about schizophrenia and homelessness. As one person said, 'Before I joined this project I used to always blame people for being homeless.' Another said, 'I realized that people diagnosed with schizophrenia have the same wants and needs as everyone, and the same as for homeless people, that they have a right to a home. I am grateful to have my own home – I don't want to be homeless and I really have empathy for those who are. They're entitled to have a place.'

Some people struggled with concerns about whether they really deserve all that they have when so many others in similar situations have nothing. As one person said, 'I had a problem with a sense of entitlement to what I have, me being on AISH and other people are not. Sometimes I have to kind of battle with that sense of entitlement to what I have. There seems to be a really big gap, and it just doesn't seem right that other people are out there who could qualify for AISH but aren't getting their needs met.' Another said, 'I guess I wonder why I'm worthy and others are not. We all should be worthy. And it made me feel guilt, like when I go out and there's people who stand on the side of the road with their signs, "There's no room in the shelter tonight." My heart breaks. And I'm thinking, I could be one of those. I'm one pay cheque away….' Another noted, 'I feel humbled that I finally have a place to live and I think of all the people that don't. Thirty-four hundred people in Calgary and going up.'

Taking part in the project also brought many rewards. One person said, 'The photovoice, what it did bring to me was a great appreciation for the loving home that I live in with my mom and it made me more grateful for the family support I have received from my mom. She's my principal caregiver and it developed greater closeness between myself and my mom and my sister who also has schizophrenia.' Another person said, 'I think we gained more than we put into it. All we had to do was take a camera and take pictures, and it took like ten, fifteen, twenty minutes. But the results are forever. They're put into a great format that everyone can see. I personally gained more and the reward was sevenfold compared to what I put into it.' Another person noted, 'It meant that I made a difference in participating in our group environment and in team spirit to contribute to some of the pictures that we had. The final product was something else.' And finally, one person said, 'It is so empowering, the photovoice. It made me realize that having a stable home is responsible for my mental wellness and all the beautiful things I am involved in and the beautiful people and colleagues that are part of my life.'

Conclusion

Through their photographs and discussions, the group explored the connections people diagnosed with schizophrenia make between their homes and their mental well-being. Group members concluded that people diagnosed with schizophrenia need stable housing that supports their desire for independence and their need for safety, spirituality, and connection to community. They highlighted positive aspects of home that contribute to their stability and pointed out that having choices about companionship with family, friends, and even pets contributes to good mental health. They also defined home in terms of their social connections with community groups, and on a broader scale, saw home as including physical surroundings such as parks and the zoo, which they find meaningful as places for contemplation and rest, something that is essential to their well-being.

The goals of photovoice as set out by its founders and proponents suggest that the political and social implications of projects such as this are of primary importance. However, all such projects must begin, as ours did, with a focus on the experiences of the people involved in the project. In our case, the project began as a personal statement about the meaning of home to the participants. Through taking photographs and thinking and talking about the meaning of the photos, group members developed new insights into the meaning of home for them personally. This was the first step in developing the project as a way to advocate for change to policies on mental health and housing. Presentations of the project at various conferences and distribution of the poster to numerous community organizations have, we hope, had an impact in raising public awareness of these issues, the first step in achieving social change.

In choosing to participate in the project, group members took on a degree of vulnerability. But the project also reinforced for them that they can contribute to research that informs social change, so participation in the project also reduced their level of vulnerability. Through their photographs and stories, the members of the project team expressed their views regarding an issue of great importance to them and explored ways that they could make a difference for themselves and for others. Inclusion in this research contributed to a sense of hope and optimism that they could in fact work their way out of the dependence/independence paradox.

6 Taking Action: Spreading the Word (Dissemination)

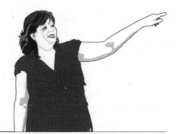

WITH LAURIE ARNEY

'I feel as a group we're heard when we go out and do our readers' theatre presentation or show our video. We have been given a platform. Compared to where we started, we have changed people's minds and people's opinions. So we have made a difference.' —Michele Misurelli

In this chapter, I describe how the research group members became involved in public discourse about schizophrenia and homelessness. We have told the stories of our interview participants and the story of our research process in a number of ways that don't fit neatly into traditional academic modes of disseminating research results. These include readers' theatre dramatic performances, a documentary film, an illustrated poster book, a travelling exhibit based on the poster book, and a project website (http://callhome.ucalgary.ca). In addition, we have been able to get a fair amount of media coverage – Michele and I have been interviewed several times on CBC radio in Calgary and she and other group members have been interviewed for various newspaper and television stories. All these forms offer the opportunity for a group of people who are generally silenced to speak directly to mental health professionals, housing service providers, and the general public about their treatment and housing experiences. This is something that would be inconceivable without the research context, as these are people who have limited opportunities to make a public statement and who are typically constrained by their need for services from making a private statement directly to their service providers.

Our twice-monthly gatherings around the table in the meeting room of the Schizophrenia Society, our personal interviews among group members and with people outside the group, and our group discussions about the meanings of the stories we collected were rewarding for everyone involved. But the rewards of these private activities pale in comparison to the rewards of taking part in public discourse. By advocating publicly for the inclusion of people diagnosed with schizophrenia as partners in decision-making about their own lives and demonstrating the abilities and strengths of people diagnosed with schizophrenia, the people in our group took action to help others with schizophrenia. They also experienced in powerful ways the potential of what they have accomplished to move them beyond the dependence/independence paradox. I discuss this in detail in the next chapter, but for now I offer a discussion of the use of alternative genres in academic research, a description of our dissemination activities, and some reflections on our successes and challenges in reaching audiences. I draw heavily on Laurie's journal entries – she is really the co-author of this chapter.

Alternative Genres for Disseminating Research

The genres we have used are a far cry from the usual academic modes for publishing research. Academic journal articles, academic conference presentations, and peer-reviewed books published by academic publishers are the genres that bring the most professional rewards to academic researchers. Funders of research typically want to see the research they have supported published in such peer-reviewed venues. This expectation has limited the ability of academic researchers to address audiences other than academic ones and to involve non-academic co-researchers and research participants in dissemination. However, this is changing. In our case, HRSDC and SSHRC's interest in and willingness to fund what is variously known as knowledge mobilization, knowledge translation, or knowledge transfer has encouraged us not only to publish in the traditional academic modes but also to move far afield from these modes and produce the genres we discuss in this chapter. Knowledge mobilization has been defined somewhat colloquially as 'getting the right information to the right people in the right format at the right time so as to influence decision-making.'[1] Our goals are even broader than this, as we hope also to influence societal attitudes towards people diagnosed with schizophrenia and to contribute to change in how they are treated.

I first became interested in alternative genres as a way to disseminate research when I saw Ross Gray's compelling and moving theatre productions based on his research with people who have cancer.[2] *Handle with Care* is based on research interviews with women who have metastatic breast cancer; *No Big Deal* is based on research interviews with men who have prostate cancer. These plays present a series of vignettes that dramatize various aspects of the lives and experiences of people with cancer.[3] I have no background at all in theatre, but I was intrigued, as performance seemed to offer a way to address the vexing ethical and political problems of representation and voice that I was struggling with in the presentation of our research.

These problems of representation grow out of the so-called 'crisis of representation' that overtook the social sciences in the mid-1980s. This 'crisis' involved a growing awareness that the descriptions constructed by academic researchers in their academic journal articles were just that, descriptions, representations, versions of social worlds produced by and for academics. Some scholars began to reject the traditional realist agenda in the social sciences that purported to discover 'truths' about social worlds and report them to readers. According to these critics, traditional realist approaches 'privilege the researcher over the subject, method over subject matter, and maintain commitments to outmoded conceptions of validity, truth and generalizability.'[4] It was no longer possible to maintain the primacy of the 'author evacuated' text,[5] in which an invisible author is but a conduit for transmitting the 'reality' of the world under study to readers.

Searching for ways to acknowledge and address the political implications of and the power relations inherent in traditional academic forms, a number of scholars in the last twenty years or so have advocated the incorporation of personal narratives and the use of genres not traditional in the academy as a way to address, if not resolve, these issues of representation.[6] This has resulted in a wide variety of forms of representation for research, including poems, plays, ethnodramas, short stories, memoirs, personal histories, fiction, creative nonfiction, photographic essays, personal narratives and essays, fragmented or layered texts, and transcriptions or dramatizations of everyday conversations, as well as dramatizations of interviews and dramatic, staged, or improvised readings.[7] These forms involve the researcher/writer in a conscious and reflexive way as a participant in the research process and as the constructor of the representation that results from this process. The attraction of all these forms is that they 'declare a reality but simultaneously reveal it as make-believe.'[8] They allow researchers to both break with and continue the ethnographic tradition of representing the lives and experiences of others. Researchers now have the opportunity and obligation to make conscious choices in forms of representation that take into account the ethical and political issues of representation. There is no one best way to represent research. Instead we can 'savor variety in our forms of representation.'[9]

Representation 'does far more than communicate about a subject; it simultaneously creates forms of relationship'[10] between researchers and audiences. While traditional academic forms of representation often produce a distant and hierarchical relationship between researchers and audiences, I am seduced by alternative genres for presenting research, as I believe they can reduce the distance and increase a sense of connection between researchers and audiences. When we expand our modes of expression, we expand the number of people who can join in the 'dance of understanding.'[11]

The genres we have chosen in our projects provide more accessible and clearer public explanations of research than is often the case with traditional academic texts. Our work does not use traditional academic conventions and it contains no technical jargon, both of which are generally barriers to dissemination to a general audience (and sometimes even within the academy). Our various genres therefore offer a more engaged relationship with audiences as they address audiences on an emotional, not just an intellectual, level. Both researchers and audience members participate in the work in a more embodied way than is possible with traditional academic genres, making the material more powerful and more memorable. Our modes of presentation provide a much richer sense of the people we studied and offer the audience 'multiple places to stand in the story, multiple levels of emotionality and experience to which they can connect their own experiences in the world.'[12] Because of the impact on audiences, we believe that our modes of dissemination offer the potential for social change. Social change does not happen quickly – it is 'earthworm work.'[13] It involves preparing the ground for change, moving the earth one tiny piece at a time, until the right moment arrives, enough earth has been moved, and change actually takes place. Engaging audiences in the ways we have done performs just this kind of earthworm work, one audience member, one poster book reader, one mind at a time.

A tension exists in the performance of research such as ours, as the performance always takes place on at least two levels. The original storytellers narrate and perform their stories during the research interviews. The researcher-performers then re-narrate or re-perform when they select material from the interviews and present the stories. The researchers-performers make the material into a public story through the performance, and in our case also through the construction of the film, poster book, and exhibit. I believe that as the adapters of others' stories, researchers have an ethical responsibility to understand the people who have shared their stories, to understand the meaning of their narratives to them, and to present them in a way that respects them and their stories. The fact that most of the people who worked on our projects share at least some of the experiences of those who were interviewed makes it likely that this has happened in our projects. But, as the crisis of representation has taught us, we can never get to reality. We are left always and only with representations. The best we can do is to be aware that public representation, whether through performance or any other means, is a political act that has real consequences for real people. If we think of these alternative genres as being not so much about description of the experiences of the people under study as about connection with audiences, then we can give up the search for 'accurate' representation and instead focus on communicating something about those experiences to raise awareness, encourage compassion, and promote dialogue.

Scripts/Performances

Our first efforts at non-traditional dissemination were our readers' theatre performances. Readers' theatre is a minimalist style of theatre with no (or very simple) sets or costumes. Scripts are used openly in performance.[14] It was first developed as a way to make literature more accessible to young people. Our use of readers' theatre overlaps with forms of populist theatre, variously called guerrilla theatre, theatre of the oppressed, forum theatre, or community-based theatre, in which the goals include community building, fighting oppression, and changing power relations in society. Although we certainly have emancipatory goals, we do not think of ourselves as a theatre group. Instead we see ourselves as researchers drawing on novel presentation modes as ways to enable the people who were fully involved in carrying out the research to participate equally fully in the dissemination of the results. Our scripts draw on data generated in our research interviews and are structured using the frameworks and ideas we developed in our data analysis. Unlike some of the examples I cited above, our performances always describe our research process as well as the results of the research.

In our first project, the idea to do a readers' theatre presentation came from Michele, who had experience with this format in a short play that the Schizophrenia Society had constructed a few years earlier. That play, called *Starry Starry Night*, dramatizes scenes in the life of a man diagnosed with schizophrenia and his family members. Except for Michele, the people in the first project had not taken part in performances of *Starry Starry Night*, but they were aware of it and had some idea of what such a performance might involve.

We followed a similar procedure for constructing the scripts in both projects. First we compiled a list of 'good' excerpts from the transcripts. This was done by a few of the group members who went through the transcripts and highlighted every piece of text that described a situation, experience, or emotion that they thought they might want to include in the presentation. The whole group then went through the 'good' excerpts, making choices and whittling the list down to a manageable number. In each project, we built the script around the analytic framework we had developed – in the first project, good and bad experiences with medical professionals, and in the second, dilemmas of care and control. In both projects, I took the selected material and, based on the discussions in the group, organized it into a script using the interview excerpts as the primary material and inserting some explanatory material to make the whole thing hang together. The group members then suggested changes to the script and I made the revisions. We began by wanting to be completely faithful to what the original speakers had said but soon realized that it was more important to capture the spirit of what had been said rather than expose ourselves to the danger of tripping over awkward constructions in performance. Editing continued as we prepared for our presentations, with group members changing the text slightly to make it easier to read or to make it sound more natural. In our performances, members of the group sit in a row of chairs in front of the audience holding their scripts. Each person stands when it is his or her turn to read and then sits down again. We use no props or costumes. A short version of a script that combines material from both projects can be found in appendix C. The longer scripts from each project can be found on our website.

Early in the process of putting together our presentations, some members of the group expressed concern that taking part in presenta-

tions would require that they be identified publicly as having schizophrenia. They feared that this might expose them to further possibility
of stigmatization. Although I stressed throughout the process that taking part in the research did not require anyone to take part in the presentations, when the moment came, they were so proud of what they
had accomplished that everyone in the first project and all but one
person in the second project took part. A discussion period after each
performance gives group members the opportunity to speak directly to
the audience, which often includes people they see as having authority
over them. This has been perhaps the most liberating aspect of doing
the presentations. People who had been extremely reluctant to speak
publicly have found themselves able to step up to the microphone to
answer questions and even challenge or contradict statements made by
audience members.

To date, our performances have been seen by hundreds of mental
health professionals in a variety of health care and community settings.
We have also performed at academic conferences in Winnipeg, Toronto,
Edmonton, Vancouver, and Calgary. When we perform in Calgary, all
the members of the group take part. For the trip to Winnipeg, we were
able to afford to send only me, Michele, and Mary. We asked the Schizophrenia Society of Manitoba to find four Winnipeggers diagnosed with
schizophrenia to take part. We had a one-hour rehearsal, presented to a
completely packed room, and received a standing ovation. For a trip to
York University in Toronto, Laurie and Monique accompanied me. We
adapted our presentation so that the three of us could read it. Laurie's
journal gives a sense of what our presentations were like.

*Laurie's Journal, 17 September 2002. At our first presentation, I hadn't quite
recovered from my hospitalization. I was quite glad we had rehearsed. We presented to medical professionals and community members. When I looked out into
the audience I saw the social worker who had helped me in the hospital. It made me
nervous, as she seemed to recognize me. I felt lots of support from the other members in the group. We did very well with our presentation. We even spoke to the
press. Later there was an article in the* Calgary Herald *about our presentation.
The audience was very interested and after we presented our findings there were
lots of questions from community members. Dr Barbara Schneider then asked if
there were any medical professionals who had questions. There was just silence
until the social worker who had advised me in hospital said, 'I don't think anyone
here wants to admit they are a medical professional.'*
Laurie's Journal, 3 & 4 October 2002. Schizophrenia Conference, Edmonton.

This was quite an experience for our group. We were all very nervous. We did our presentation twice in one day. The conference was large; the audience was all people interested in schizophrenia. There were medical professionals, representatives from drug companies, family members, researchers, and on and on. We presented in the later half of the day in workshop type format. After we did our presentation and recommendations, we broke the audience up into smaller groups. We then went into the audience and talked with them. For me the whole experience was very empowering, as it put me on a level playing field with persons who oftentimes had power over me. I felt heard where it might make a difference some day in the treatment of people suffering from schizophrenia. To top it all off the experience was fun, with the group all travelling together in a rented van with Dr Barbara Schneider driving. We stayed the night in a very classy hotel and met people from all walks of life.

Laurie's Journal, 17 January 2003. *8:00 a.m. Foothills Hospital. We presented to doctors' rounds. I don't know how I managed to make it through this presentation, as mornings are really difficult for me. Dr Barbara Schneider said we all did great.*

Laurie's Journal, 17 April 2003. *Presenting to a group of Psychiatric Residents. One doctor after hearing us speak said words to the effect that he will never be able to treat his patients quite the same way he used to. Seeing us stable and being able to voice our concerns made us so real to him, like everyday people. They fed us lunch and everything.*

Laurie's Journal, 18 May 2006. *Dr Barbara Schneider, Monique Solomon, and I met to work on the script for our first presentation at York University. We did a run-through of Housing: Issues of Care and Control and the photovoice presentations for errors, timing, and reading. We had to make changes, as sometimes the written word is not the same when it is spoken. It is strange that the spoken word seems to need to have more clarity and often sentence structure has to be changed. Also Dr Barbara introduced a chart that worked really well. It was good to be part of this process. I often could help keep the point of view of the group in mind. I felt honoured because I would be representing the research participants from the Schizophrenia Society.*

Laurie's Journal, 3 June 2006. *The York University Experience. The adventure to Toronto, where I grew up. Coming back, nothing was familiar. I was here to do the presentation with Dr Barbara Schneider and Monique Solomon. I was nervous and excited. Our rooms were in residence. I thought they were great even through we had to share washroom facilities with the rest of the women on the floor. I started to think how great it would have been if I had had the chance to go to university and live in residence when I was young. I wondered what my life would have been like if I did not have schizophrenia.*

I was quite nervous about our presentation and practised my part every day until Sunday. The presentation went quite well, though I did not realize how much speaking I had to do. It was quite a challenge. I talked too fast. I also have to remember to breathe at the end of sentences and new paragraphs. There were a lot of questions asked. Some people wanted to see more of the dark side of housing instability. That was not what our presentation was about. We were highlighting the needs for those with mental illness acquiring and maintaining housing stability. Also bringing to light the unique challenges they face with issues of care and control. I felt we did get through to a lot of the members of the audience. I had a number of people come up and talk to me afterward. A lot of people also like seeing a presentation with a more positive slant, with answers and recommendations that would improve the housing situations for the mentally ill.

Someone asked me what I think of the 'Disability Culture.' It left me speechless for a moment. I said something like, 'Sometimes when you disclose, you can take on more than you are prepared for. You can get stuck and have trouble moving through all that having a disability does to you. It can sometimes be quite hard to focus on your abilities and have the strength to move forward.' I have to find more information about this.

Laurie's Journal, 20 September 2006. *The research group did our performance at the Starfish Café in Calgary. This was the night Tom Everrett filmed the group for the presentation part of the film. We had rehearsed enough now that we did really well for this presentation. We had a very large audience and that helped give that needed nervous energy. I noticed that for me the fear factor was gone. I felt comfortable with what I had to say and rest of the group sounded great too.*

Laurie's Journal, 6 October 2006. *We presented our work at the Schizophrenia Conference in Edmonton. We did really well presenting twice to groups of twenty to twenty-five people. There was a lot of input from the audience, who had similar concerns as our group.*

Laurie's Journal, 17 November 2006. *We did our presentation at a Homeless Conference at Grace Baptist Church in Calgary. The presentation went really well. The press interviewed Michele and me afterwards. Michele handles herself like a pro – she really gets her message across. We did get in the news. I am hoping we made some impact on how having schizophrenia affects housing stability and causes homelessness.*

Laurie's Journal, 12 January 2007. *Psychiatric Rounds. We presented at the University of Calgary medical school theatre. We were linked by video to the Rockyview Hospital and Fort McMurray. One of the comments I wanted to make note of after we did our presentation was that one of the doctors said, 'Advocacy is not a billable service for doctors.' We presenters did get on a bit of a vent about* *the control aspect of care. We also talked about addictions. I commented that it is important to get the person housing first and then work on the addictions.*

In 2007, I stopped being the main organizer of performances and Michele took over. The Schizophrenia Society received a small grant to pay Michele to do this and she invited any interested members of the Unsung Heroes support group to take part in performances and be paid for their participation. This gave members of the Unsung Heroes who did not take part in the research projects the experience of talking publicly about their experiences, something that, I hope, offered them some of the benefits of participation that are articulated by the members of the research group in the next chapter.

Documentary Film

The making of the film was the least participatory of our endeavours. A method of participatory video production exists,[15] similar to photovoice, that enables community members to visually represent their reality through making their own videos. However, we were all somewhat worn out by the activities we had undertaken in the projects over a period of many years and did not have the energy to add yet another activity that would involve group members in making their own video. So we hired Tom Everrett, at the time a graduate student in the Faculty of Communication and Culture at the University of Calgary, to make the film. Tom has an undergraduate degree from Ryerson University in film and television and had been involved in the housing project in a very peripheral way for about a year before we made the film.

The film is based primarily on interviews with the members of the group about how they got involved in the project and what it was like for them to do the research. Tom and I took our camera and a few rented lights, and over a period of three days, went to the home of each member of the research group, where we conducted and filmed an interview. We also filmed the first performance of the housing script. Tom then cut together excerpts from the interviews and the performance into a twenty-nine-minute documentary film. At various times in the construction of the film, I showed a rough cut to the group members. They made some suggestions – for example, that we dramatize the situation of homeless people by adding shots of people sleeping under bridges. However, we were unable to do this because we did not have ethics clearance to film people who were not involved in the project as research participants. We have shown the film at numerous community events and conferences. It has also been seen by audiences all over the world as people from many countries see it at conferences and take it home to use in their classes and communities. Laurie describes our film presentations in her journal:

Laurie's Journal, 8 December 2006. This was the debut of our film at the University of Calgary. There was standing room only and my family was there. I missed a couple of meetings, so it was the first time I saw the film from beginning to end. Everyone in the film did wonderfully. Tom Everrett made sure that the most important messages were brought forward and somehow drew all the threads of the different personalities to the forefront. Afterwards, the group went to the front of the room. There was a standing ovation at the end of the film. It was quite overwhelming.

Laurie's Journal, 5 January 2007. Our film was shown to Dr Barbara Schneider's Communication Class. Jamal and I attended to participate in presenting the film and for the discussion part after. There was a good discussion after the film, especially when we talked about the wellness that was brought to the group members by being involved with this project. I talked about being able to talk to university students, and how it helped me to feel I belonged. Now I have learned how to more fully balance my life. I am now focusing on staying well and working part-time. One student said the film was like a breath of fresh air.

Laurie's Journal, 9 January 2007. The Marda Loop Justice Film Festival. Our film 'Hearing (Our) Voices' was shown. Jamal, Mary, Michele, and I went to the front of the audience to answer questions. Michele of course was incredible, didn't skip a beat. I mentioned that we presented our film to university students, and that those working in the field were also concerned about the homeless situation. I said, 'I saw the news, and corporate Calgary is on board to find solutions to wipe out homelessness.' Then I heard that Michele had been in the news too, so I gave the mike back to Michele and said, 'Talk!' I did talk about my building and how it was the best available for persons with mental illness, and that the care was there when needed, and the support for being independent. Jamal talked about educating people about schizophrenia. Mary talked with someone who asked, 'How do you let care givers know when you want to be more independent?'

Laurie's Journal, 23 January 2007. Alberta Mental Health Board (AMHB) presentation and movie. We were linked by video to Edmonton, Ponoka, and Lethbridge. The president of the AMHB was in the audience in Edmonton and gave very positive feedback, saying how important this work is, 'Especially to hear the voice of the consumers.'

Laurie's Journal, 24 May 2007. Presentation of film 'Hearing (Our) Voices' at Central Community Mental Health Clinic in Calgary. After the film Barbara and I answered questions. It was a little uncomfortable at times. One psychiatrist asked if housing issues were going to be addressed at the federal level and if not, said there was no sense talking about anything. Another therapist said how they were all wounded as they were like sponges absorbing our pain. I felt kind of bad for that therapist.

Poster Book

Our poster book makes the research available in yet another way, particularly to people diagnosed with schizophrenia. The book is immediately accessible – readers just have to open it for a few minutes to be intrigued and to see the point of what we are doing. This is in contrast to our film, which, although it is easily portable, requires the right equipment and a willingness on the part of the audience to sit down and watch for twenty-nine minutes, something that can be a barrier to our ability to reach audiences. Although I was not specifically looking for a way to address this, our poster book in fact solved exactly this problem.

Construction of the book was an intensely collaborative process. The illustrations and book design were created by Colin McDonald. Over the year that we worked on the book, the group met monthly to work on the text that would go into the book and to discuss how the illustrations should look. Colin knew almost nothing about schizophrenia when he started working with us, so these meetings were essential for him to begin to understand the goals that participants had for the book and to create drawings that would reflect their experiences in the mental health and housing systems. We started with the text from the readers' theatre presentations of both research projects and spent several meetings editing it down to the absolute minimum that would convey the essence of the speaker's experience without losing anything. Colin spent his time during these meetings sketching participants, generally getting to know them and their concerns, taking notes of their conversations and stories, and occasionally pointing out that the text was still too long. At several points during the year, he and I put together a mock-up of the book and made a photocopy for each person in the group. They made suggestions for the drawings and layout that Colin then incorporated into his design. The book was printed by a local print shop and has been distributed across Canada and worldwide. It is also available for downloading on our website. Laurie describes our work on the poster book:

Laurie's Journal, 5 January 2007. First meeting for illustrated poster book. The group met with the graphic artist, Colin. He designed our poster, 'Searching for Sanctuary.' He suggested the book have eight main parts. That led to an open discussion as to what the group would like those themes to be. Some suggestions were rent, income, AISH, support from family and friends, the system, and abuse experienced from the medical system. The last one, medical abuse, seemed to bring up a lot for some members of the group. The telling of stories of abuse under medical care seems to occupy a lot of the group's time. Dr Barbara Schneider suggested that maybe we should think about combining both our research projects for the poster book. Things to keep in mind are that the poster book should be for all audiences. We will continue to meet the first Thursday of each month to work on the book.

Laurie's Journal, 1 February 2007. Meeting for poster book. Colin presented his ideas for main topics: home, hospital, AISH, the system, transportation (walking, bus, LRT, and Access Calgary). Also themes to be covered: workplace (AISH, volunteer work, support groups), care and control (medical issues, housing, finances, meaning of home). How when we interact with our world, we have to always be grateful even when we are not feeling that way. The stories will be around six generic people diagnosed with schizophrenia (he is not sure how to make them identifiable yet). I have to laugh out loud here. I like his idea of making the people in the hospital waiting room have one large body and lots of heads. Then he wants us to tell him our stories to help with the dialogue, once he has a drawn the backgrounds and lots and lots of people.

Laurie's Journal, 24 May 2007. Meeting for poster book with Colin, Dr Barbara Schneider, and the Research Group. Colin had the text and some of the drawings laid out for the poster book. I especially liked the drawing on page 20 with the bird, the dog, and the man all looking in the same direction. The group told more stories of their experience. There was an idea of a patient streaking, with a nurse with a needle and a team of security guards running after the streaker as a theme running through the book. I thought the idea had a lot of merit.

Our first opportunity to distribute the book was at the Schizophrenia Society Christmas party. This was attended by numerous people who have been diagnosed with schizophrenia and their friends and family members. Several people immediately asked for additional copies to take to their doctors or to give to their friends who do not have a diagnosis of schizophrenia. This is our fondest hope – that people who are diagnosed with schizophrenia will use the book to change the attitudes of their doctors, family members, and others who seek to help them rebuild their lives. We also held a book launch for the poster book in

December of 2007. Pages on Kensington, an independent book store in Calgary, offered us their space to do a reading for friends, family, and others who saw our advertisements or heard Michele and me talking about it on the radio that day. Laurie describes:

> *Laurie's Journal, 10 December 2007. Our poster book was launched on December 4th, 2007. Dale, Jamal, Mark, Mary, Suzan, Michele, and I did a reading. George didn't want to read, so Michele's daughter Jennifer took his part. Dr Barbara Schneider and Colin McDonald were there to celebrate the launch too. It was inspiring as the turnout was huge and most of us had family members there for support. We had many comments about how well we all read and how important the poster book was. There was a wine and cheese buffet after the reading and the press was there also. It was the first time some of the group members saw the published poster book. We were excited to get our own copy. Myself and other members mingled with the audience and at the same time tried to get our books signed by all who took part in its making.*

Travelling Exhibit

We received another grant, this time from HRSDC, to turn the poster book into an exhibit to be shown in cities across Canada. Our graphic artist, Colin McDonald, adapted the poster book illustrations and turned them into a series of large posters that have been displayed in hospitals, treatment centres, civic centres, and libraries in various cities across Canada. Group members accompanied the exhibit to locations in Alberta to give a short reading and meet the press. This too can be seen on our website.

Taking Action

Group members are convinced of the importance of their participation in public discourse. They know that their presentations offer insight into the perspectives and experiences of people diagnosed with schizophrenia and contribute to an understanding of the medical and housing systems in Calgary from the point of view of people on the receiving end of services. The presentations also give group members an opportunity to demonstrate to audiences that people diagnosed with schizophrenia are real human beings, with the same kinds of concerns and feelings that everyone has. The responses we get at our performances and video screenings have both heartened us and discouraged us. On the one hand, we believe that our research is contributing to change in the practice of health care for people diagnosed with schizophrenia through our influence on the mental health professionals who see our performances. On the other, we have often felt frustrated by the slow pace of change and the overwhelming odds against us when confronting a large institutionalized system of care.

Heartening are the comments we received after performances for psychiatrists and residents at two Calgary hospitals. At one hospital, a psychiatry resident told us that he had seen us at a previous performance and that he had changed how he interacts with his patients as a result of hearing group members speak about their experiences. At the other, a psychiatrist who practises only in the hospital commented that he never sees patients when they are well, only when they are sick. It was something of a revelation to him to hear the group members speak so articulately and poignantly about their treatment experiences. These are just two small comments, but they illustrate the potential for change on a larger scale. We do not hear from everyone who sees our work and so cannot estimate the impact it might be having unbeknownst to us.

We have also been encouraged by comments we get from members of the general public who have seen our presentation and film. After our book launch, at which group members read some sections of the poster book, one of the people in the audience told me that he had no idea the experience would be so moving and transformative for him. Our film regularly brings audiences to tears. A woman who saw the film and read the poster book wrote to me in an email: 'As a psychology graduate, what struck me most after reading *Hearing (Our) Voices* and seeing the DVD was how little I had learned about schizophrenia during my studies. Textbooks and diagnostic manuals typically do not give an accurate picture of what living with schizophrenia truly means. The human being living with the disorder tends to be forgotten. *Hearing (Our) Voices* puts a human face on what is otherwise simply a clinical label.' While it is hard to estimate the effect this kind of response has, it seems to us that it can only be a positive step towards reducing negative perceptions of people diagnosed with schizophrenia.

On the other hand, as Laurie says about our presentations to medical professionals, 'I notice that the things they didn't want to hear, they kind of closed down to. It was hard getting across to them that some things that were happening shouldn't be happening – that this should stop. As soon as we said good things about them, that's when they keyed in. They wanted to hear what they were doing right but didn't want to hear what was going wrong.' In order to avoid alienating our audiences, we have been careful to include the positive aspects of people's experiences in all our presentations. We want to acknowledge that the people we interviewed have had good experiences in the mental health system and that people who work in the mental health system have good intentions and certainly do not set out to provide bad care. But as Laurie points out, our strategy of including positive experiences may give people who think of themselves as caring individuals a way to avoid hearing about the negative aspects of the care they provide. It allows them to think that other people may do things that are problematic but they themselves do not.

We have also been frustrated by what we see as our inability to get the attention of politicians and other people in a position to make policy changes. As Dale said, 'To a certain extent we are preaching to the converted. It would be nice to get our hands on the people who actually make the decisions.' None of us are politically savvy or connected in ways that would give us access to the ears we want. For example, Michele wrote letters about our project to people she perceived to be policy makers – the leaders of all the political parties in Alberta. But, she says, 'I haven't received anything back, so now I have to call again, and they keep putting you off. So that's kind of discouraging. I want them to see our presentation, to see our film, but it's really hard to make inroads.' Getting the attention of policy makers requires a pubic relations approach that, as researchers, we simply do not have the skills or budget for. Cindy summed up her frustration: 'I'd like to get Stephen Harper [currently the prime minister of Canada] and sit him in a room for an hour and give him a piece of my mind.' In fact, about a year after these conversations, Michele succeeded in getting an invitation from the Alberta Provincial Liberal Caucus to present a short version of our readers' theatre performance. These small successes keep group members dedicated to continuing to present their perspectives on their experiences and working to make a difference in the lives of others with schizophrenia. Earthworm work takes time and patience, and we remain confident that we have produced knowledge that, because it is different in form and content from most research in the field of mental health, makes a real contribution.

7 Where We Got To (Conclusion)

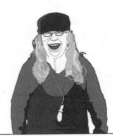

WITH CONCETTA RANIERI AND LAURIE ARNEY

'I got a job. After doing the presentations, doing a job interview isn't so daunting as it used to be. After you manage those presentations, it kind of gets you ready for a lot.' —Laurie Arney

'If I could say one thing to any other people diagnosed with schizophrenia, it is that you have a right to speak against a doctor. It's your life and you should put forth what you want. It should be a negotiation, not a one-way communication.' —Michele Misurelli

In this chapter, the group members tell the story of their participation in the research projects and describe how the projects affected their lives. In addition to creating knowledge and taking action based on that knowledge, participatory action research has a goal of empowering and transforming the lives of the people who take part. This goal has been accomplished in spades in our projects, but it has been a wonderful by-product of our research rather than something we actively set out to do. I believe this happened because the research was not just an activity designed to fill time and be 'therapeutic.' Instead the group members were engaged in something that had great meaning and importance for them. They saw the potential of their efforts to have an impact on the lives of others. Neither they nor I thought at the beginning of the impact it might have on our own lives. I confess, though, that in my darker moments, I reassured myself that if the research did not manage to have a wide public impact, if it had even a small impact on the lives of the people involved, I would be able to feel that we had accomplished something worthwhile. I am gratified that we have accomplished both.

The quotations that appear in this chapter come mainly from a focus group with the research group members conducted by Laurie Arney, one of the group members, assisted by Concetta Ranieri, at the time a master's student at the University of Calgary. The focus group was attended by all of the people who took part in the housing project except me. Laurie and Concetta asked questions during the session, and Laurie also answered some questions. They asked participants about why they had decided to become involved, how they felt about being co-researchers, how it affected them, and what they had learned. The session took place as usual for an hour just before a regular Unsung Heroes support group meeting at the Schizophrenia Society. The tape recorder was managed by Concetta and the tape was transcribed by our professional transcriber. A few additional comments in this chapter come from reflections written by some group members at a meeting quite near the end of the second project. We also include comments from people who took part only in the first project – Laurie phoned Dana and Ken to ask if they had anything they wanted to say.

Transforming the Lives of Participants

The central theme that emerged in the focus group discussion was the desire of group members to make a difference in the lives of others who have been diagnosed with schizophrenia. Claude said, 'I wanted to take part in the research to make a difference and to make my peers realize that mental illness is not a dead end. There are lots of possibilities.' Cindy felt that it would be a way to help people who struggle as she does. 'I wanted to be in the research because I like to help people and I saw it as a way to try and help my peers. It allowed me to be part of the solution, not part of the problem.' For Mark, the research was an opportunity to change the negative perceptions that limit the opportunities and affect the quality of life of those with mental illness: 'I did the research because there is terrible discrimination out there and I want to tell about the horrible things that go on with the illness, plus the stigma and the prejudice against the mentally ill.' Similarly, for Michele, making a difference meant fighting for the equality of people diagnosed with mental illness and dignifying them as human beings who deserve basic rights such as stable housing and fair treatment. Mark agreed. 'We have got to fight all the way to get rid of these inhumanities in the hospital. I think some people are really bad people, really strange, they won't listen to you. Maybe one day they'll change the way people are treated while under their care, but it might take a long, long time.'

The presentations in particular gave group members a feeling that they were accomplishing something worthwhile. They all became public speakers, able to articulate their concerns directly to people who they feel have authority over them. As Jamal said, 'I have a voice and I've been heard, and for a long time people with a mental illness were the silent minority.' For some, the presentations also had a therapeutic effect. Laurie said, 'For myself I found doing presentations, especially the Claresholm [a residential treatment centre in Alberta] presentation, brought me resolution.' Ken said, 'At the beginning I found the presentations nerve-racking, but the rehearsals and practising helped immensely. I enjoyed performing the presentations at hospitals and all the other venues. I found it empowering. I realized people in the audience were a lot like me, only most of them did not have schizophrenia.' Dana too said, 'It was all very empowering, the whole experience. We were actually getting to people and they were understanding. It empowered them too. It served both causes – the participants' and the audience's. I love the fact that it opened some doctors', nurses', and caretakers' eyes to the point where they asked questions and they listened.' George agreed. 'You really get a reward after you've done this. You see the film and listen to the people and answer the questions. I think it's a really worthwhile thing to do.' He also expressed his pride in the quality of the work done by the group members. 'We practised over and over again. We've become quite professional and highly polished. I think we've done really great.' Dana too noted, 'We improved with each presentation. We were more vocal and also started taking more pride in our appearance.' Taking part in the presentations allowed group members to validate their experience, have their concerns heard, and show what they were capable of.

The presentations also provided a good chance for people to get know each other. As Michele said, 'It was fun and I thought the trips really brought us closer as a group.' If our presentations were in Calgary, we usually had lunch together before or after the presentation. If we went out of town, we travelled together. Michele recalled a trip we took during our first project to a treatment centre about a hundred kilometres from Calgary. We rented a van and set off down the highway. Michele describes: 'A steel piece that was on top of the van we were travelling in kept banging against the roof of the van and it was driving poor Dr Schneider crazy. So we stopped in High River and bought duct tape and duct taped the van back together. It was kind of a bonding experience with the duct tape.' We had many other bonding experiences as our work became better known and we were invited to do more presentations and film showings.

The research projects also gave group members a feeling of being valued. Claude said, 'I feel I belong. I belong to the group, and I also have been able to enhance my skills in terms of helping to run a few groups and give input. I'm almost relied on in some ways.' Being relied on is something that many people diagnosed with mental illness do not experience. Typically they are recipients rather than providers of anything. Being able to contribute something that others see as valuable and even necessary promoted a real sense of membership. They also talked about the friendships they made in the group and described the unique social support network they established. Several said that what brought them together was the fact that they were people with similar experiences working towards a common cause. As Jamal explains, 'Working as a team made me realize about relationship building and what it's like to work together with people with a common illness and the issues facing us.' Because they shared common experiences, they could also empathize with each other about the trials each has faced. As Dana said, 'There was such team spirit. We were there for each other. There was such comradeship among us, lots of pats on the back.' Suzan said, 'I am proud of these people. They are my friends.'

We also just had fun together, something that is often missing from the lives of people diagnosed with schizophrenia. We had good laughs during our meetings and did social things together outside our group meetings. As Laurie said, 'I especially enjoyed our outings for dinners, the social interactions, and learning more about everybody in a different way outside of our concerns with the research. Just people talking about our everyday concerns and what we've been up to. I realized how diverse we are in all our activities.' Mary commented, 'Many aspects of the project were fun – always a joke to lift the weight of our contemplation. I found it great to see the positive, cooperative working beside people that I don't ordinarily see.'

The feeling that they were doing something important kept group members coming to meetings even when they found it difficult to do so. And certainly, although the group members have very positive feelings about their experiences, everything did not go smoothly all the time. Participating in the research was often very emotional for group members. Some found it difficult to listen to the stories told by the people they interviewed. They could not help but empathize with them but felt powerless to do anything to help them. As Cindy said, 'I wanted to do something constructive. I wanted to kick ass, to make somebody do something, and I didn't know how. So I got frustrated and angry.' The interviews also reminded them of their own difficult life experiences. But as Laurie said, although letting out bottled-up emotions was difficult, it helped them to deal with those deep feelings and find some closure. 'Sometimes the stories did get over-emotional and they affected me. But at the same time I realized I was not alone in my hurt and pain, and finally I was talking to other people who knew what I was talking about. Though some of us had a hard time, as time went on it seemed to help us deal with a lot of our own emotions that had piled up over the years.' The presentations too were emotionally difficult but gratifying. Mary noted, 'I found hearing the material again [in the presentations] was just overwhelming, and I didn't speak much afterward because I was afraid to. But I was really hoping for the response we got. People seemed to listen in earnest and ask good questions.' Despite all the emotional challenges, group members felt strongly that the stories of the people they interviewed needed to be told, and that is what kept them going. As Dale explains, 'I guess you can get depressed with some of the stories, but you have to push that to the side so that you can bring those stories out for other people to understand.'

Group members also said they learned a lot from the project. Dana noted, 'It opened my eyes to what was important, and I realized what was important to me was not necessarily important to someone else and vice versa.' Mary found that 'It has been a learning experience – digging deep for emotions, showing our true feelings and insights to the research material. Like how rough others had it and appreciation of their strength to endure the worst and get better situations for themselves. It was eye-opening, as well as giving us some satisfaction about getting our voices heard.' Dale commented, 'I think it really helps because you get to see what other people have experienced through their eyes. I think that's more important than talking to somebody who is an academic or a politician or somebody who has never been involved in that situation.' Jamal too says he learned something: 'My participation in this research made me realize how ignorant I was about the homeless issue. It has opened my eyes.'

Several group members described their increased confidence in dealing with their various medical encounters and their increased expectation that their concerns will be addressed. Dana said, 'The presentations helped us learn how to speak out. We also learned to question situations and realize when we were entitled to more.' Cindy said she had learned to be more assertive. She told a story in which she described a situation in a walk-in medical clinic where she waited to see a doctor for what seemed like forever. She finally went up and asked the receptionist how long she would have to wait. It turned out that somehow her name had not been put onto the list and her file had not been put into the pile. The receptionist remedied this and Cindy was seen very soon after. This may seem to readers like a very ordinary thing to do, not requiring any special skills or confidence – to confirm that you are actually on the list and ask when it will be your turn. But to Cindy, having the wherewithal to ask a medical person, even a receptionist, a very simple question is a big step forward. This speaks to the kind of treatment that people often receive in the mental health system in which they are expected to be docile, unquestioning recipients of treatments and are scolded or coerced when they ask questions or object to their treatment. As Michele explained, 'When a doctor says something, I always thought that you couldn't talk back or have an opinion.' However, after participating in the research, she has learned to be more assertive. Now she says, 'If they say something I don't like, I tell them. It's my life, you're not making decisions for me. It's my life, you can give me suggestions but nobody's controlling my life but me. My life could have been so different.'

Other group members also noted that they now are able to speak more openly to their doctors about their individual needs. George says he is better able to speak to his psychiatrists about his concerns. 'I've become not self-enclosed.' Laurie provided a specific example of how she became more active in interactions with her psychiatrist. 'I found communicating with my doctor and making changes to the type of supports I wanted, that now I have more of a voice. Just recently I was having a problem with cholesterol, and the psychiatric medication I'm on was contributing to that. So I went in and talked to my psychiatrist and we're doing a little bit of adjustment to my medication. It is good to be able to contribute in those important decisions concerning my medical care.'

The confidence they have gained through their participation in the research projects has also assisted many of them to contribute in other meaningful ways to society. Michele has had several opportunities to speak about the research on radio and television. Jamal has written articles about the research projects that have appeared in the *Calgary Herald* and the *Schizophrenia Digest*, among others. During the research, Cindy wrote letters about the poor treatment she had received in the hospital, one of which was published in the *Schizophrenia Digest*. She read this letter at a forum of Calgary Health Region mental health workers. When asked about what it was like for her to read the letter out loud, she said, 'I was surprised, I just started reading. I was a little nervous when I started and just bam I didn't care who was there, who was listening, I just wanted to say my piece and I was fine.' The experience in the research helped Laurie to land a small teaching job where she earns her own income. She explains, 'I think doing the presentations really helped me not to be afraid to talk to people that I think have power over me. Now I can talk to them just as a regular person and not have that fear. It helped me to have confidence to go on to teach Continuing Education courses in crochet.'

Another theme in the focus group was group members' perception of my role in the projects. I felt a bit embarrassed to be on the receiving end of their praise and found this material extremely difficult to write. In reviewing an early draft of this chapter, group members felt strongly that what they had said in the focus group about me and what I brought to them were not sufficiently highlighted. Laurie came to my office one day and explained the importance of including this information in the chapter not only because it was important to group members, but also so readers could see the impact of my approach on their lives. Laurie wrote this section.

Laurie: When the research group members found out that I was helping Concetta with a chapter in the book, they let me know how wonderful it was to work with Dr Barbara Schneider. They said I had to make sure this got into the book. I feel the same way – it was wonderful. Dr Barbara has a unique approach; she does not seem to see the disabilities. She makes everyone feel important. She sees what you are capable of, she believes in you, and the next thing is, you find yourself believing in yourself. These sentiments are not only my own, but were shared by all group members during our focus group.

I think what Dr Barbara did most for us was to see us as capable human beings first and foremost. None of us ever felt like research specimens. Dr Barbara made us feel like valuable equal contributors in all phases of the research. Jamal explains: 'What I like about Dr Schneider is she's a listener. She's not judgmental and she gives everybody a fair chance, and she treats everybody as equals. She's a wonderful and remarkable and caring person to work with. I enjoy working with her. She's down to earth and humble and she's so easygoing and relaxed.' Dale also emphasizes the respect and worth we all felt in her presence in his statement, 'She's good, she's very patient, she listens to what you have to say and she doesn't make a lot of judgments about anybody.' Furthermore, this respect extended beyond our research encounters, as she treated us as important individuals even in instances of everyday social interaction. Cindy remembers a time when she saw Dr Barbara as she was running some errands. 'I even bumped into her once going into the grocery store and she stopped to say hello and talked to me for five minutes before going inside.'

What was really important about our relationship with Dr Barbara was how different it was from our other encounters with professionals. Even though she too is a doctor, a doctor of communication, our encounters with Dr Barbara were very different from our encounters with medical doctors. She saw something in us most professionals do not. At each meeting, it felt as if Dr Barbara knew what we were capable of before we even did. Michele's comment highlights this. 'She had a vision in her mind of what she thought we could accomplish. She has insight, she has foresight, and she has a gentleness. She treated every one of us like we were the most important person in the room.' Mary agreed: 'We know she took to heart what we were saying, because we could tell through the compilation of material that she found the important parts of it.'

Dr Barbara Schneider is an incredible role model for all professionals working with individuals with mental illness. She has a way of making us feel comfortable and accepted. She cares about each person as an individual. Through the research projects she taught us how to speak out and advocate for others, which in turn taught us how to advocate for ourselves. Because of all this, she shows by example how professionals can make a difference in how people diagnosed with schizophrenia are treated. In Dana's words, 'We love her. She invoked pride and power in us and more. She taught us how to fish.'

For me too, participating in these projects has been a transformative experience. When I started the projects, I knew almost nothing about schizophrenia. My acquaintance with it was similar to that of many people – when I was growing up, I knew that one of my mother's friends had a son who was diagnosed with schizophrenia. But I really did not pay much attention and understood nothing of the experiences of either mother or son. When my own son was diagnosed, I was thrown into the strange and unnerving world of the mental health system, where I met psychiatrists, social workers, nurses, case managers, and other grieving parents. But still I knew only one person diagnosed with schizophrenia, my own son, and had no sense of what the future might hold.

Doing these projects allowed me to get to know many people diagnosed with schizophrenia, some of whom have been living with this diagnosis for many years. Through our work together, we became a supportive community, something that benefited me as much as it did them. Sharing a small corner of their lives through our research meetings and social events enabled me to see the variety of abilities, skills, and strengths they possess. This and the passage of time have helped me to come to terms with having schizophrenia as a permanent fixture in my family life. Our work showed me that I could be both a mother of a person diagnosed with schizophrenia and a researcher and teacher and that I could bring these together in fruitful ways. Although I cannot say that I have truly achieved acceptance, I no longer think, even subconsciously, that I can make schizophrenia go away. Coping with schizophrenia is my son's job in life, not mine. I can provide support only from a distance because he wants the same independence from coercive family or professional control that you have read about in the preceding pages.

So You Want to Do Some Research

Before we conclude our narrative, we offer some advice to people wanting to carry out research similar to ours. A number of helpful resources exist written by mental health service user researchers such as Alison Faulkner and Peter Beresford.[1] We do not need or want to replicate what they and others have done. As they and almost everyone else who writes about service user involvement in research acknowledge, this kind of research is rewarding but also demanding and requires commitment on the part of everyone involved to make it successful. Our story has illustrated the rewards but also the hurdles and challenges that research of this kind must confront, so here I provide a brief discussion of what I regard as key issues followed by advice from some of the members of our research group.

Perhaps most important is the involvement of service users in every aspect of the research, right from the beginning. Without this, research runs the risk of returning to the control of professional researchers with service users relegated to advisory or consultative roles. Such involvement is key to avoiding tokenism or watering down of the service user voice in the research. Involvement must be understood outside the usual terms of professional research. Some service users want to lead and carry out their own research, but not all want this level of responsibility. And not every service user who wants to be involved can contribute in the same way. Researchers, and here I refer to both professional and service user researchers, must make space for the inclusion of a wide range of people with varying abilities, valuing and incorporating the contributions that each person can make, and not dismissing people for the contributions they are unable or choose not to make. Much is lost if only the most able, confident, and assertive service users are involved.

No one 'right' way exists to 'do' service user involvement in research. Flexibility and a willingness to negotiate every aspect of the research are the keys to success. All researchers must be willing to engage in negotiations about how to work together and how to proceed with the research. Professional researchers must be careful not to assert, consciously or unconsciously, their professional authority or their assumptions about knowledge and must be open to unexpected questions or directions in the research. Flexibility is required in adjusting the research plans in response to developing understandings of the research problem. Critics might see the requirement for this kind of flexibility as compromising the 'quality' of the research, implying that when service users are not involved, this kind of adjustment doesn't happen. In fact, most research involves a series of compromises as reality or new information intervenes to disrupt the best-laid plans, and this is no more true of research that involves service users than it is of other kinds of research.

The need for approval from institutional ethics review boards may seem to be a barrier to the ability of service users to carry out research. However, the process of applying for such approval forces researchers to think carefully about their goals and plans. Although in participatory research it can be hard to say exactly how a project will unfold, I have found the process of articulating the research plans (to the degree that it is possible) to be extremely helpful in moving the project planning forward. I have also appreciated the advice of ethics committees, particularly when they have jogged me about things that I should have thought about but had not.

Service user involvement in research inevitably increases the time needed to complete research and demands patience on the part of all who are involved. Negotiations about how to carry out the research, training of participants to carry out various research tasks, and discussions of data during the analysis phase, to mention but a few issues, are all likely to slow the process. Professional researchers must be prepared for it all to take much longer than they expect, and both professional and service user researchers must be in for the long haul. But it is in the long haul that the rewards are to be found, rewards that far outweigh the challenges in the doing of the research.

Members of the research group responded with the following comments when I asked them what advice they could offer to others. Jamal's advice was offered to professional researchers. He suggests they need to have 'a sense of compassion, caring, and empathy, and an open mind to the topic being researched. In choosing a topic for research, they should consult with the co-researchers on what topic is important to them. They should work closely with the co-researchers in trying to bring about change to situations where improvements are needed.' Laurie also had advice for professional researchers. 'Having a leader who gives a lot of responsibility to group participants is important. I felt like there was no tight control over the group, and everything just kind of unfolded. There was always group consensus when it came to decisions, yet participants were free to participate to the extent that they wanted. I liked that there was the option of anonymity.' Laurie also had advice for service user researchers. 'It is important for you to know that you are the only one that can contribute your story. Your story added to the other participants' stories becomes of great value. Be open to trying new experiences like doing interviews and being interviewed. Listening was really important and also learning a lot from the feedback from audiences and understanding different points of view.' Michele sees the importance of making sure that co-researchers make a commitment to a certain level of involvement (in our case, twice monthly meetings for at least two years) and that they have a strong desire to make change. She also thinks that a project needs 'a facilitator who keeps people on track, doesn't let the project get bogged down, and gets outside help for the group when needed. Dr Schneider found someone to help us learn how to do focus groups and got people to help when we got stuck with the data analysis.' She also thinks that it is important for the group to engage in team-building activities, such as our dinners together.

Readers will have noticed that the members of the Unsung Heroes addressed me in various ways: Dr Barbara Schneider, Dr Schneider, Dr Barbara, but rarely Barbara, the name I asked them to call me. At the beginning of the projects, I think they regarded me in much the same way they regarded the many other professionals in their lives – as someone they must be polite to or risk losing something. They may also have had a sense that others would expect them to address me respectfully as 'Dr.' As group members became more confident about asserting their ideas and wishes, our relationships changed. I was no longer the unquestioned leader, and different people took the lead at different times. But it would be disingenuous to suggest that we became equal partners. I remained the only person in the group without a mental health diagnosis, and the only person with a PhD and a university job. As I noted in chapter 2, power relations are the most challenging aspect of carrying out this kind of research, and their forms of address to me illustrate how hard it is to overcome status distinctions. But I believe that, over time, 'Dr Barbara Schneider' went from being a sign of deference to being a term of endearment mingled with respect. And I changed too. I came to know, admire, and respect my co-researchers, who taught me just how much people diagnosed with schizophrenia have to offer society.

Epilogue

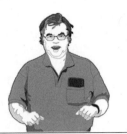

We are at the end of our narrative, at least for now. The story will never end in the lives of the people who took part in the research. We are all forever changed by the experience and take those changes with us into the rest of our lives. We have told a story of ability and accomplishment, and we believe that we have achieved the three interrelated goals of participatory action research to generate knowledge, take action to implement that knowledge, and have a transformative effect in the lives of the participants. We are perhaps most proud to have joined the small but growing number of people who are doing research that involves mental health service users as co-researchers.

We generated knowledge that makes a significant contribution to understanding the experiences of people diagnosed with schizophrenia in the medical and housing systems. Our projects contribute to what has been described as a 'sparsely inhabited'[1] intersection of schizophrenia research and qualitative methods through the use of interviews and focus groups to obtain access to the experiential realities of people's lives. But more important, by integrating people with a diagnosis of schizophrenia themselves as co-researchers, we kept the focus on their concerns throughout the projects and produced knowledge that would not have been available even in other kinds of qualitative studies.

Our analysis of how care, control, and communication interact in the lives of people diagnosed with schizophrenia has contributed to the literatures on relationships between people diagnosed with schizophrenia and their medical practitioners and on housing for people diagnosed with schizophrenia. We show that open and collegial communication is central to mitigating the dilemmas of care and control. The lives of people diagnosed with schizophrenia are affected by a number of aspects of treatment relationships (i.e., diagnosis, medication, information, and support), but all of these are embedded in communication, in both the informational and relational senses. Communication is vital also in relationships with housing service providers, something that is rarely mentioned in the housing literature.

Our research also provides support for the housing first model. This model asserts that people should have choices and that they should not be forced to live in circumstances in which they must continually prove their worthiness for housing, as in the linear continuum model. Group members are adamant that housing should be provided as a basic human right, not contingent on treatment compliance or sobriety, and support those who advocate for the provision of permanent housing in the community in which people are supported but are relatively free from control exerted by housing and other service providers.

We took action to improve the lives of people diagnosed with schizophrenia by telling as many people as we could about our research through various non-traditional modes of dissemination. Group members became public speakers, able to directly address people who have an effect on their lives and on the lives of others like them. They 'helped the cause' with every readers' theatre performance and film screening. They also spread the word in the poster books and the exhibit. We know through responses to our work that some service providers have changed how they interact with people diagnosed with schizophrenia, and we can only hope that this change will spread like a ripple to others working in the field of mental health.

And finally, we all experienced the transformative impact of participating in projects of this kind. Involvement in research is the first step, but having frequent opportunities to share the research with service providers, politicians, and the general public is key in enabling mental health service users to regain a sense of themselves as contributing members of society. Through generating knowledge and taking action to improve the lives of others with schizophrenia, group members helped themselves to achieve a sense of self-determination and empowerment in spite of continuing to struggle with experiences of schizophrenia. In focusing on helping others, they found new meaning and purpose in their own lives, tapped into their own potential for growth, and began to emerge from the dependence/independence paradox.

Storytelling is a social act – stories must be heard by listeners in order to become public stories. The storytellers in our projects are a group of people typically marginalized and silenced, routinely discredited by their diagnosis of schizophrenia as legitimate speakers in any realm, but particularly in their dealings with care-giving professionals and institutions. Taking a narrative approach has enabled them to offer a counter-narrative to the old medical story of schizophrenia in which people are told to expect to be permanently disabled and unable to achieve anything in life. Instead, as you have seen, the people involved in these projects are extremely articulate about their experiences and about the meanings their experiences have for them. They are well able to identify when they have been treated in inhumane ways and to ask to have their essential humanity and personhood recognized in their treatment and other social interactions.

In the end, our work is really about how people diagnosed with schizophrenia can claim full and equal citizenship as participants in and contributors to society.[2] Our work illustrates that it is not the limitations experienced by individuals that determine whether they can participate fully as citizens. Rather it is the dominant stories that create barriers in society that exclude some as unworthy of full citizenship. People diagnosed with schizophrenia may need support to achieve full participation, but it is in providing this support that society holds a mirror to itself and shows that it values the essential humanity of every member, including those diagnosed with schizophrenia. We hope, through all of this, that we have persuaded you of the necessity and value of including people diagnosed with schizophrenia in research, in decision-making about treatment, and in public discourse about schizophrenia.

Eight years ago we started our journey, taking small steps, most weeks taking a new step, some weeks taking a step backwards. Getting involved, committing ourselves to a collective path, and sticking with it has led us to places we never imagined could be ours, but that we have made truly our own.

Appendix A
Interview Questions

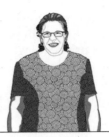

Schedule of Questions for the Communication Project

When were you diagnosed?
What medication are you on?
What is your medical history?

How do you relate to your psychiatrist?
How does your psychiatrist respond to you when you complain about
   side effects?
How do you feel in the presence of your psychiatrist?
Can you talk to him/her on a personal level?
Do you like your doctor/psychiatrist? Does he/she like you?
Do you understand your doctor/psychiatrist?
Would you like to be able to choose your doctor?
How well informed are doctors about treatments and side effects?
Do you know if you are on a high dose or a low dose?
How often do you see your doctor?
How long does he/she spend with you in clinic? How long would
   you like him/her to spend with you?
How many residents have you been a guinea pig for?
Do you have any positive experiences with medical professionals you
   can tell me about?

Tell me about your hospital experiences. Do you usually get in easily
   when you need to?
What caused you to be brought to hospital?
How much time does your nurse spend with you helping you get
   better?

Did they talk about you in your hearing? Do they talk more among themselves than with you?

Did you get privileges when you got better (in hospital)?

Describe your follow-up program after you were released from hospital.

Were you involved in a support group?

How do medical professionals respond to emergencies?

What is your status with police, fire department, paramedics?

How is your relationship with your pharmacist?

Do you feel institutionalized or criminalized?

Has your psychiatrist told you what your diagnosis is?

Was the illness explained to you? If so, how was it explained? How do you feel about that?

Did you see any visual aids (films, overheads) or written material?

What support or information did your family get?

Do you know about AISH? How did you find out about it?

Tell me about aspects of your life: exercise; work history and experiences; diet, nutrition, weight; side effects of medication; interaction with peers; addictions to alcohol, food, caffeine, tobacco, street drugs and other meds. How does alcohol interact with your meds?

Can you afford your medication?

Have you been made fun of or bullied?

How do you manage interpersonal relationships? Do you have the same friends as before?

What are your dreams and goals for yourself?

Do you think you will get better?

How would you like to see psychiatry (and other medical professions) change?

How do you feel now?

Is there anything else you would like to tell us?

Schedule of Questions for the Housing Project

1. Questions about Diagnosis and Life Experience with Schizophrenia

When were you diagnosed with schizophrenia?

Tell us about your experiences with schizophrenia.

Were you hospitalized? How long?

Did your hospitalization ever affect your housing situation?

Was there conflict or tension in your family because of your mental illness?

Does your family understand your mental illness?

Did you get information about where to go for help?

2. Questions about Housing Circumstances

How long were you/have you been homeless?

How did you become homeless?

What led up to you becoming homeless?

Where were you living before you became homeless?

What was your mental health status before/during the time you were homeless?

Did you get medical treatment? What was it like being homeless? What was your experience?

How did you feel? How did people treat you? What were your fears? Who were your friends?

Did you experience abuse and violence?

How did you take care of personal needs such as food, sleep, hygiene?

What time of year was it when you were homeless?

Were you threatened by gangs or police?

Tell us about a place you have lived. Pick one: Describe what it was like. What was the neighbourhood like? Who lived with you?

Where do you live now? How did you get the apartment? How did you get the damage deposit? How do you pay for it?

3. Institutional Connections

Was welfare or AISH a barrier to getting housing?

Was a social worker available to you in hospital?

Were social workers in hospital helpful to you in dealing with housing?

What help did you receive? Which agencies, family? Tell us about someone who really helped you.

Were you ever turned away from housing?

Were there barriers to getting housing: damage deposits, references, security, hookups?

4. What Does Home Mean to You?

Where would you like to live? What would be your ideal circum-
stances?
What kind of supports would help you to get and stay in housing?
Has it been helpful to you to have social workers in your building?
What kinds of supports are important to you? Money management,
social and recreational activities, on-site counselling or social work-
ers, life skills training, on-site clinical services?
Do you feel safe in your present situation?
What do you worry about?

What would have to happen for you to be able to stay in your housing?
What does home mean to you?
Is there anything we forgot to ask you or more that you want to tell
us?

Appendix B
Calgary Herald Articles about the Project

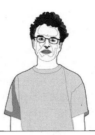

Article by Barbara Schneider Printed in the *Calgary Herald*, 22 February 2007

Numerous articles about homelessness in Calgary have appeared in the news in recent months. While it is heartening to see attention being paid to such an important social issue, notably absent from the discussion are the voices of people who have themselves been homeless. Long-term solutions to such a complex problem are elusive and likely to remain so without attention to the experiences and views of those who are most affected.

Over the past two years, I have been leading a participatory action research project on housing for people diagnosed with schizophrenia. Participatory research involves as co-researchers people who have experienced the problem being studied. In this project, nine members of the Unsung Heroes peer support group for people diagnosed with schizophrenia from the Schizophrenia Society of Alberta, Calgary Chapter took part as co-researchers. Together we interviewed thirty people who have schizophrenia and have been homeless. My comments here reflect the conclusions that the research team drew from their own housing experiences and from the interviews they conducted. People diagnosed with schizophrenia are a subgroup of people who are homeless, but the issues they raise in our study illustrate the complexity of the problem of homelessness.

According to the people in our research, they experience a continual tension between care and control in their relationships with their service providers. While service providers have good intentions and want to help them, care, it seems, never comes without a dark underbelly of control. Service providers have authority and power over those they serve. A relationship intended to be positive, empowering, and enabling is at the same time controlling and disempowering.

The people in our research say they need, want, and appreciate the housing services and other help they receive from family members, mental health professionals, government agencies, and housing and other social service providers. But, to receive that care, they must submit themselves to intrusive surveillance and coercive control over many aspects of their lives.

But it is even more complex. The people we talked to are ambivalent about control. They don't really like it, but sometimes they appreciate control that prevents them from doing things that have led to housing instability in the past. And sometimes they make a rational decision to walk away from housing services that intrude too much into their lives.

For the people in our study, control is encapsulated in the word 'compliance.' Compliance is kind of a dirty word – it means that you do exactly what the doctor, social worker, or psychologist tells you, or you risk losing housing and other services. Compliance is probably not a bad thing in an acute illness. But with a chronic illness like schizophrenia, it means a lifetime of suppressing your own wants and needs in order to maintain your relationships with housing and other service providers. And it means a lifetime of being grateful even when things are not really as you would like them to be.

What is the solution? How can people who are homeless receive the care they need without having to submit to unwanted control? Don't ask me. Ask the people who know best – those who are on the receiving end of housing services.

The research team members produced some recommendations for promoting housing stability. Here is a little bit of what they have to say. They want to be treated with respect and dignity, something that is sadly not always the case. Although they are mentally ill and may be living on a disability pension, 'do not ask us to expose our whole lives.' They want to be listened to when they express concerns about the housing and other help they are receiving. They want service providers to work with them to help them make choices, but not tell them what they have to do. 'We do not want to be forced to live the way you think we should live.'

Discourse about homelessness is dominated by experts who speak about and for those they think are too sick, troubled, or downtrodden to speak for themselves.

To those who truly want to solve this problem: Please, make it your responsibility to listen to the voices and views of people who are or have been homeless. Without them, you cannot find long-term solutions to the problem of homelessness.

To see the full list of recommendations please go to the research project website: http://callhome.ucalgary.ca

Article by Jamal Ali Printed in the *Calgary Herald*, 9 March 2007

In her article, 'Listen to those who have been homeless,' *Calgary Herald*, 22 February 2007, Dr Barbara Schneider, research project leader, mentioned the importance of listening to the voices and views of people who are or have been homeless.

As one of the co-researchers afflicted with schizophrenia, this project has proven to be an enlightening experience for me. I attended my first Unsung Heroes meeting at the Schizophrenia Society of Alberta, Calgary Chapter in October 2004. I was so impressed with the warmth and support displayed by my colleagues towards one another at that meeting. What followed was my regular attendance at successive meetings.

My involvement in the research project Housing for People Diagnosed with Schizophrenia: Dilemmas of Care and Control is a unique experience for me. It was overwhelming at first, because it is so different from the type of research that I was familiar with during my four years of study at the University of Calgary (1976–80): library research on topics of interest for my term papers in the Social Science and Humanities undergraduate courses.

Participatory research is about human interaction. There existed a relationship of sharing as the research team listened to those participants afflicted with schizophrenia and their experience with homelessness during the interview process.

I admire the participants for their willingness and courage in sharing their experiences during the interview process. Their story reflects the stark realities of homelessness. I came close to tears when I heard the heartbreaking stories of their experiences. Overall, the research team was very moved by their stories.

Our contributions to the research clearly refute the notion that people with a mental illness are unproductive members of society. We have demonstrated that we are capable of pursuing a challenging project despite our medical condition.

What is so impressive about us is the spirit of cooperation that we have instilled among ourselves and the research leader in making this project a reality and a success. Schneider has commended us for our eagerness, determination, and courage. Her confidence in her co-researchers was instrumental in our success.

I consider it an honour for my colleagues and me to be working together with Schneider on the participatory action research project. She is truly a remarkable person to work with. She is a caring and wonderful person.

Homelessness is detrimental to the mentally ill's state of mind. This difficult situation worsens the mental health of those afflicted with schizophrenia, bipolar, and other forms of mental disorders.

Accessibility to affordable housing creates a healthy environment for the mentally ill. A roof over their heads and a place that they can call their own play a vital role in the effective management of their illness.

What has the research done for me? Since I have always been fortunate to live with my parents, the research has transformed me from an indifferent person to a compassionate individual.

Before the research, I never paid attention to the plight of the homeless individuals afflicted with a mental illness. I would often blame them for their housing situation. This research has greatly dissolved my ignorance regarding this issue.

My participation in the research project was a learning experience. I have developed a greater understanding and awareness of the difficult situation of homelessness experienced by the mentally ill. As a result of this understanding and awareness, I have developed a sense of sympathy and empathy for those who have gone through this ordeal and those who are currently in this situation.

What's the intent of the research? At some point in the future, the research team hopes to present its research to influential authorities at the local and provincial level. Our objective is to bring awareness to the housing crisis facing the mentally ill in Alberta. Our hope is that the research will convince the decision makers to help in the process of building more affordable housing.

We have done a number of research presentations at various venues: the schizophrenia conference held in Edmonton in October 2006, the Calgary Health Region's conference on homelessness held in Calgary on 17 November 2006 and the Alberta Mental Health Board in Calgary on 23 January 2007, etc. The impact on the audiences was powerful. They were moved and inspired by our presentation.

It's my hope that this research will open up the hearts, ears, and minds of society. Society has to make affordable housing a priority. It's their moral right and social responsibility.

Appendix C
Script of a Readers' Theatre Presentation

This script can be read by any number of participants. When we read it, one person acts as the 'narrator.' He or she reads the introductory paragraphs and all the bolded material. Other participants take turns reading the bulleted passages.

Schizophrenia: Hearing (Our) Voices
Dilemmas of Care and Control

Welcome to our presentation today. It is based on research that was carried out by a group of people diagnosed with schizophrenia under the guidance of a university professor. We all worked together as co-researchers on two participatory action research projects. The first project was on communication between people diagnosed with schizophrenia and their medical professionals. The second was on housing for people diagnosed with schizophrenia. We chose the topics for the research and carried out interviews and focus groups with people like ourselves who have schizophrenia and have experienced housing instability.

The main theme of our work is the tension between care and control in our relationships with medical and housing service providers. People who care for us want to help us. But they also have authority and power over us. A relationship intended to be positive, empowering, and enabling is at the same time controlling and disempowering.

The words you are about to hear come from our interviews and focus groups with more than thirty people who have schizophrenia. We do not speak for all people diagnosed with schizophrenia, only those who took part in our research. We have many positive things to say about our experiences with medical and housing service providers. We also have some negative things to say. We offer this presentation not to be critical but in the hope that you will understand the experiences and point of view of people diagnosed with schizophrenia.

The System
People in the medical and housing systems have helped us to rebuild our lives.

- I've been lucky. I have a treatment team that cares and really listens to me.
- With the way the old system was, the psychiatrist had all the control. Now the pendulum is swinging back to the middle, where we're gaining some control back.
- It was a big breakthrough when I was on the disability pension. Having a steady income has helped me to keep paying the rent.

Service providers want to help us, but they also want to control us.

Dilemma: We must always be grateful for the help we receive, even when things are not really as we would like them to be. We are afraid of asking for even small changes for fear that we will lose what we have.

- Once you're in the medical system you can't get out of it. If you try to get out of the system, then you don't get your meds or your doctor, and you need those things.
- If you want to break away from the label, they say, 'Well then, we won't take care of you. You're uncooperative and you're uncompliant.'
- It's almost like an additional disease, just trying to understand all the agencies, and what they want from you, and what you're supposed to do, and what your diagnosis is.

Family
Help from family can make all the difference.

- Without parental units that care, I would have been homeless many, many times. Your life skills are hindered and humbled as a result of your mental health challenge.

- My sister helped me get my own place. She taught me how to look after money, how to do the house-cleaning, and how to look after myself properly.
- My sister bought a condominium for me. She pays the mortgage and I pay the condo fees and utilities. I look after her cat when she is out of town and she does the repairs and painting.

Many people diagnosed with schizophrenia have conflict with family. Even help and support can seem controlling or disempowering.

Dilemma: How do we maintain our independence and at the same time know when to ask family or friends for help?

- Since I was adopted, there have been problems in the home. When I became older, I just started running away.
- Family likes to believe that you're doing well. It makes them feel good, so they're not open to listening.
- My siblings can't accept that I have schizophrenia. They are afraid of me and don't include me in social events. I feel abandoned and forgotten.

Hospital
Good hospital care can help us recover and get back to our homes and work.

- My doctor was doing something with my medications and I was really upset. So he explained it all to me. I said, 'I understand why you made the change.' And he said, 'Thank you for understanding.'
- My doctor asked me just one question: 'What do you need to feel better?' And everything came into place.
- I think the best thing that I've learned is to be assertive. If you don't want to do something, tell them.

We are not cases. We are people. We are not just something to be managed.

Dilemma: They want us to comply with treatments, but they don't tell us why, or listen to us, or treat us with respect.

- When I first went to the hospital, my doctor did not tell me my diagnosis. The student doctor took me aside and said, 'We think you have paranoid schizophrenia.' For cancer or heart attacks, they always tell you, 'You've had a heart attack, you've got cancer, you've got leukemia.' Only with mental illnesses, they won't tell us.

- They think we don't notice, but we know when we are being treated inhumanely. If I was a heart attack victim they would cater to my every need. But I'm in the psych ward. They ignore you at the nurses' desk.
- It's just one-way communication, from them to us.

Identity
We have had to learn to live with schizophrenia.

Dilemma: To get the care we need and want, we have to accept the label, person with schizophrenia. But once we have the label, we can't get out from under it in any area of our lives.

- When I first learned that I had schizophrenia, I thought, is that something from the dark ages? Are there asylums where I will be committed and never get out of?
- I still have a hard time dealing with the fact that, yes, I have schizophrenia. I'm still in denial and I probably always will be, because who wants to be this way?
- Why are you worthy and I am not? We should all be worthy. We are still beautiful, but we are treated as less than beautiful because we have slipped in our stability.
- I go to the coffee shop with my friends. They know I have schizophrenia, and they like me. We do cryptic crosswords and if I am having problems, I can talk to them. I get a real feeling of fitting in and being part of society.

Medication
Medication has helped many of us to maintain stability, but it often leads to bad physical health.

Dilemma: We are told that we are responsible for our own recovery and for making our own choices. But we are limited by what service providers think are the right choices.

- Going off medication is my greatest fear, because it's a downhill slide. I've had enough of it to realize that it's not fun. It seems fun at the time, but when you look back at it, you don't think so.

- Do I walk around crazy, or do I take the meds and put up with the weight gain, and stiffness, and blurred vision, and dry mouth, and all the other side effects?
- The medical profession calls our pharmaceuticals chemical restraints. It's really hard to explain to them how it feels when they give us too much. But it's like being tied up in certain areas of us.

Housing
Home is a place to find sanctuary.

- Home is a very safe place, where I don't have any fears or nightmares.
- I spent many nights not sleeping, wandering the streets. To go to bed and fall asleep and not worry about anything is a real treat. It's a real blessing.
- You get such a sense of self-respect when you walk into a place and you know no one is going to say, 'You shower when I say,' or 'You eat when I say,' or 'Things don't go there,' or 'You're not allowed to have those friends here.'

Getting and keeping decent affordable housing can be a challenge.

Dilemma: Should we live in supported housing with lots of help, but also rules and scrutiny? Or should we pay high rent and eat macaroni but feel free?

- If you're sick you can't keep your job. If you can't pay your rent, you can't keep your house.
- I moved into a basement suite. There were mice and mould and mushrooms growing out of the carpet and water seeping in. I trapped ten mice and threw them in the garbage. It was a dungeonous place, but I had to live somewhere.
- I have to bring my cat. A lot of people don't understand that, but she's my whole world. I just can't give her up. I live for her. So because I had a cat, I had to go into slum housing.

Recommendations
We have some recommendations for medical and housing service providers.

- It is your responsibility as medical professionals to communicate with us. We have schizophrenia and we can't always manage our interactions with other people.

- Treat us with the same respect, dignity, and kindness that other patients get. No matter how sick and unstable we may be, we are human beings first.
- Tell us what is wrong with us. If someone has a heart attack or cancer, you tell them what is wrong with them, but with mental illness, you won't tell us.
- Listen to us and respond to our concerns about side effects and about how medications affect our physical health. Our physical health is as important as our mental health.
- Don't ask us for compliance. Work with us to help us make choices, but don't force us to live the way you think we should.
- We should be able to live where we want to live. Help us realize our dream of living in our own homes in the community.
- We are living with a mental illness and are on a disability pension, but this does not mean you should ask us to expose our whole lives.
- We need a central agency for the city that knows about all the housing options for people with mental illnesses.
- Simplify the disability pension system. The paperwork required by the pension is so overwhelming, it makes you not want to work.
- Don't make us share with roommates unless we are willing.
- Provide different ways of housing people, including people with pets.
- We need rent controls and more subsidized housing. We must find the political will to have more subsidized and affordable housing.

Notes

Prologue

1 An article he wrote about the research for the *Calgary Herald*, along with one I wrote, is reprinted in appendix B.
2 In schizoaffective disorder, the symptoms of both a mood disorder (e.g., bipolar disorder or depression) and schizophrenia are thought to be present.
3 All of my work is available on my personal website: www.ucalgary .ca/~baschnei. Examples include: Barbara Schneider, 'Mothers Talk about Their Children with Schizophrenia: A Performance Autoethnography,' *Journal of Psychiatric and Mental Health Nursing* 12 (2005): 333–40; Barbara Schneider, 'Narratives of Schizophrenia: Constructing a Positive Identity,' *Canadian Journal of Communication* 28(2) (2003): 185–201.

1: Introduction

1 Barbara Schneider et al., 'Communication between People with Schizophrenia and Their Medical Professionals: A Participatory Research Project,' *Qualitative Health Research* 14 (2004): 562–77.
2 Peter Reason and Hilary Bradbury, 'Introduction: Inquiry and Participation in Search of a World Worthy of Human Aspiration,' in *Handbook of Action Research: The Concise Paperback Edition*, ed. Peter Reason and Hilary Bradbury (London: Sage, 2006), 1.
3 Other excellent sources of information about participatory research include Orlando Fals-Borda and Muhammad Anisur Rahman, eds., *Action and Knowledge: Breaking the Monopoly with Participatory Action Research* (New York: Intermediate Technology / Apex, 1991); Peter Reason, 'Three

Approaches to Participative Inquiry,' in *Handbook of Qualitative Research,* 1st ed., ed. Norman K. Denzin and Yvonna S. Lincoln (Newbury Park: Sage, 1994), 324–39; Stephen Kemmis and Robin McTaggart, 'Participatory Action Research: Communicative Action and the Public Sphere,' in *Handbook of Qualitative Research,* 3rd ed., ed. Norman K. Denzin and Yvonna S. Lincoln (Newbury Park: Sage, 2005), 559–604.

4 See Michael Oliver, 'Changing the Social Relations of Research Production?' *Disability, Handicap, and Society* 7 (1992): 101–14; Gerry Zarb, 'On the Road to Damascus: First Steps toward Changing the Relations of Disability Research Production,' *Disability and Society* 7 (1992): 125–38.

5 See Fabricio Balcazar et al., 'Participatory Research and People with Disabilities: Principles and Challenges,' *Canadian Journal of Rehabilitation* 12 (1999): 105–12; Peter Beresford, 'A Service-User Perspective on Evidence,' in *Choosing Methods in Mental Health Research: Mental Health Research from Theory to Practice,* ed. Mike Slade and Stephen Priebe (New York: Routledge, 2006), 221–30.

6 Community mapping refers to the involvement of community members in creating visual representations of their communities to answer questions about circumstances and resources in the community. For example, it might be used to map available mental health care facilities in a community and transportation links between them. See John L. McKnight and John P. Kretzmann, 'Mapping Community Capacity,' in *Community Organizing and Community Building for Health,* ed. Meredith Minkler (New Brunswick: Rutgers University Press, 2006), 158–72.

7 Because our research was carried out by people who have the same kinds of life experiences as those they were studying, our approach also fits well into what some authors call autoethnography [e.g., Bryant K. Alexander, 'Performance Ethnography: The Reenacting and Inciting of Culture,' in *The Sage Handbook of Qualitative Research,* 3rd ed., ed. Norman K. Denzin and Yvonna S. Lincoln (Thousand Oaks: Sage, 2005), 411–42; Norman K. Denzin, *Performance Ethnography: Critical Pedagogy and the Politics of Culture* (Thousand Oaks: Sage, 2003)]. Personal narratives, both of the researchers and of other participants in the research, are central to autoethnography. In general, 'the living body/subjective self of the researcher is recognized as a salient part of the research process' (Tami Spry, 'Performing Autoethnography: An Embodied Methodological Praxis,' *Qualitative Inquiry* 7 (2001): 711). This allows researchers to 'connect the personal to the cultural' (Carolyn Ellis and Arthur P. Bochner, 'Autoethnography, Personal Narrative, Reflexivity: Researcher as Subject ' in *Handbook of Qualitative Research,* 2nd ed., ed. Norman K. Denzin and Yvonna S. Lincoln [Thousand Oaks: Sage,

2000], 740) as a way to encourage cultural awareness and social change. Researchers fold their own experiences into the experiences of others by studying 'those biographical moments that connect us and our private troubles…to the larger public culture and its social institutions' (Norman K. Denzin, *Interpretive Ethnography: Ethnographic Practices for the 21st Century* [Thousand Oaks: Sage, 1997], xviii).

 8 For a comprehensive bibliography of such research see Michael Turner and Peter Beresford, *User Controlled Research: Its Meanings and Potential. Final Report* (Brunel University: Shaping Our Lives and the Centre for Citizen Participation, 2005).

 9 Jean Campbell and R. Schreiber, *In Pursuit of Wellness: The Well-Being Project* (Sacramento: California Department of Mental Health, 1989).

10 Cheryl Forchuk, J. Jewell, R. Schofield, M. Sircelj, and T. Valledor. 'From Hospital to Community: Bridging Therapeutic Relationships.' *Journal of Psychiatric and Mental Health Nursing* 5 (1998): 197–202. Canadian Nurses Association, *Preparation for Community Living: The Bridge to Discharge Project* (Ottawa: Canadian Nurses Association, 1996).

11 Larry Davidson et al., 'Phenomenological and Participatory Research on Schizophrenia: Recovering the Person in Theory and Practice,' in *From Subjects to Subjectivities: A Handbook of Interpretive and Participatory Methods*, ed. Deborah L. Tolman and Mary Brydon-Miller (New York: New York University Press, 2001), 163–79.

12 Jonathan Delman, 'Consumer-Driven and Conducted Survey Research in Action,' in *Towards Best Practices for Surveying People with Disabilities*, ed. Thilo Kroll, Juliana Cyril, Paul O. Placek, and Gerry Hendershot (Hauppage, NY: Nova Science, 2007), 71–87.

13 Diana Rose, *Users' Voices: The Perspectives of Mental Health Service Users on Community and Hospital Care* (London: Sainsbury Centre for Mental Health, 2001); Diana Rose, 'Collaborative Research between Users and Professionals: Peaks and Pitfalls,' *Psychiatric Bulletin* 27 (2003): 404–6.

14 Alison Faulkner and Sarah Layzell, *Strategies for Living: A Report of User-Led Research into People's Strategies for Living with Mental Distress* (London: Mental Health Foundation, 2001).

15 Jim Walsh and Joan Boyle, 'Improving Acute Psychiatric Hospital Services According to Inpatient Experiences: A User-Led Piece of Research as a Means to Empowerment,' *Issues in Mental Health Nursing* 30(1) (2009): 31–8.

16 Jan Wallcraft, Beate Schrank, and Michael Amering, eds., *Handbook of Service User Involvement in Mental Health Research* (London: Wiley, 2009).

17 Angela Sweeney et al., eds., *This Is Survivor Research* (Ross-on-Wye, UK: PCCS Books, 2009).

18 Budd Hall, 'Introduction,' in *Voices of Change: Participatory Research in the United States and Canada*, ed. Peter Park, Mary Brydon-Miller, Budd Hall, and Ted Jackson (Toronto: OISE Press, 1993), xvii.
19 Fisher proposed the narrative paradigm as an alternative to the rational paradigm that he says has dominated Western thought for several centuries. Central to the rational paradigm is the idea that people are basically rational beings who make decisions on the basis of logical arguments. The world consists of logical puzzles that can be solved through rational analysis and argumentative reasoning. Rationality is determined by how much we know and how well we argue. This perspective underpins much of the thinking in many academic disciplines, including mental health research. The dominance of the rational paradigm means that knowledge that is based on logical argument is valued more highly than knowledge that is not. Fisher believes that the assumptions of the rational paradigm limit our understanding of reason and rationality by separating logic from everyday discourse. He describes the rational paradigm as 'but one way to tell the story of how persons reason together' ('Narration as a Human Communication Paradigm,' *Communication Monographs* 51 [1984]: 3). Fisher does not deny reason and rationality as understood in the rational world paradigm, and does not argue that the narrative paradigm should supplant the rational. Rather, he seeks to reconstitute rationality to offer another story about 'truth, knowledge and reality.' His very broad definition of narration as 'symbolic action – words and/or deeds – that have sequence and meaning for those who live, create, or interpret them' (*Human Communication as Narration: Towards a Philosophy of Reason, Value, and Action* [Columbia: University of South Carolina Press, 1987], 58) offers an alternative to the notion that communication must be argumentative to be considered rational and paves the way for a perspective that includes values and emotions, as well as aesthetic considerations, as legitimate aspects of knowledge.
20 Fisher, 'Narration as a Human,' 15.
21 Fisher, *Human Communication*, 24.
22 Walter R. Fisher, 'Narration, Reason, and Community,' in *Memory, Identity, Community: The Idea of Narrative in the Human Sciences*, ed. L.P. Hinchman and S.K. Hinchman (Albany: State University of New York Press, 1997), 307–27.
23 Fisher, 'Narration, Reason, and Community,' 318.
24 Fisher, 'Narration, Reason, and Community,' 323.
25 Fisher, 'Narration, Reason, and Community,' 309.
26 Fisher, 'Narration, Reason, and Community,' 309.
27 See Larry Davidson, *Living outside Mental Illness: Qualitative Studies of*

Recovery in Schizophrenia (New York: New York University Press, 2003); Michael F. Greene, *Schizophrenia Revealed: From Neurons to Social Interactions* (New York: W.W. Norton and Company, 2001).

28 For example, individuals were thought to be possessed by the devil or by witches. They were in the grip of mysterious powers. They had 'worn-out' nerves, too much blood flowing to the head, or a surplus of strength and energy. Now we no longer think of the devil and witches or of nerves and energy. But even over the course of the twentieth century there have been a number of ways of understanding schizophrenia: as a result of unconscious conflicts; as a creative response to an untenable family situation; as a sane response to an insane world; as a result of poor parenting or schizophrenigenic mothers; as a response to being labelled.

29 This phrase was made famous by Nancy Andreason, *The Broken Brain: The Biological Revolution in Psychiatry* (New York: Harper and Row, 1984).

30 See for example R.D. Laing, *The Politics of Experience* (New York: Pantheon, 1967), and Thomas Szasz, *The Myth of Mental Illness: Foundations of a Theory of Personal Conduct* (New York: Harper and Row, 1974). See also David Pilgrim, *Key Concepts in Mental Health* (London: Sage, 2005), for an excellent overview of how this debate is understood today.

31 Linda J. Morrison, *Talking Back to Psychiatry: The Psychiatric Consumer/ Survivor/Ex-Patient Movement* (New York: Routledge, 2005), describes the history of this movement and its work in advocating for change in how people with mental illnesses are regarded and treated in the mental health system. This movement has adopted the disability rights movement slogan, 'Nothing about us without us.'

32 See Pilgrim, *Key Concepts*, 132.

33 There exists some debate about whether schizophrenia has existed throughout human history or is a more recent human development. E. Fuller Torrey, author of a widely used manual for parents (*Surviving Schizophrenia: A Manual for Families, Consumers, and Providers* [New York: HarperCollins, 2006]), believes schizophrenia appeared in the Middle Ages but he acknowledges that others believe it has always been part of the human condition.

34 Greene provides a fascinating and accessible discussion of schizophrenia (*Schizophrenia Revealed: From Neurons to Social Interactions* [New York: W.W. Norton and Company, 2001]).

35 Greene, *Schizophrenia Revealed*.

36 Manitoba Schizophrenia Society, *The Truth about Schizophrenia: Why You Should Change Your Thinking about Youth's Greatest Disabler* (Winnipeg: Manitoba Schizophrenia Society, 2000), 8.

37 Courtney M. Harding and James H. Zahniser, 'Empirical Correction of Seven Myths about Schizophrenia with Implications for Treatment,' *Acta Psychiatrica Scandinavica* 90 (supp. 384) (1994): 140–6.
38 E.g., Patricia Deegan, 'Recovery: The Lived Experience of Rehabilitation,' *Psychosocial Rehabilitation Journal* 15(3) (1988): 3–19.
39 See, for example, Delman, 'Consumer-Driven'; Harding and Zahniser, 'Empirical Correction'; Patrick A. McGuire, 'New Hope for People with Schizophrenia,' *Monitor on Psychology* 31(2) (2000) http://www.apa.org/monitor/feb00/schizophrenia.html (accessed 21 January 2008); RoAnne Chaney, 'The Value of Consumer Involvement in Medicaid Managed Care,' Centre for Health Care Strategies Brief, http://www.chcs.org/usr_doc/consumer_involvement.pdf (accessed 21 January 2008).
40 Davidson, *Living outside Mental Illness.*
41 Deegan, 'Recovery.'
42 For example, Luc Ciompi, 'Catamnestic Long-Term Study on the Course of Life and Aging of Schizophrenics,' *Schizophrenia Bulletin* 6 (1980): 606–18; Luc Ciompi, 'The Natural History of Schizophrenia in the Long Term,' *British Journal of Psychiatry* 136 (1980b): 413–20; Larry Davidson and Thomas H. McGlashan, 'The Varied Outcomes of Schizophrenia,' *Canadian Journal of Psychiatry* 42(1) (1997): 34–43; Courtney M. Harding et al., 'The Vermont Longitudinal Study of Persons with Severe Mental Illness, I: Methodology, Study Sample, and Overall Status 32 Years Later,' *American Journal of Psychiatry* 144(6) (1987): 718–26; Courtney M. Harding et al., 'The Longitudinal Study of Persons with Severe Mental Illness, II: Long-Term Outcome of Subjects Who Retrospectively Met DSMIII Criteria for Schizophrenia,' *American Journal of Psychiatry* 144(6) (1987): 727–35.
43 See, for example, www.mhrecovery.com; www.power2u.org/articles/recovery/new_vision.html.
44 Davidson, *Living outside Mental Illness,* 46.
45 Nora Jacobson and Dianne Greenley, 'What Is Recovery? A Conceptual Model and Explanation,' *Psychiatric Services* 52(4) (2001): 482–5.
46 See, for example, a number of articles about doctor/patient communication in Teresa L. Thompson et al., *Handbook of Health Communication* (London: Laurence Erlbaum Associates, 2003).
47 Harding and Zahniser, 'Empirical Correction,' 143.
48 W.P. Hornung et al., 'Collaboration with Drug Treatment by Schizophrenic Patients with and without Psychoeducational Training: Results of a One-Year Followup,' *Acta Psychiatrica Scandinavica* 97(3) (1998): 213–19; M. Oehl, M. Hummer, and W. W. Fleischhacker, 'Compliance with Antipsychotic Treatment,' *Acta Psychiatrica Scandinavica* 102(6) (2000): 83–7; Sian

Llewellyn-Jones, Gill Jones, and Peter Donnely, 'Questions Patients Ask Psychiatrists,' *Psychiatric Bulletin* 25(1) (2001): 21–4.

49 Faulkner and Layzell, *Strategies*; Rose, *Users' Voices*; Anna Hackman et al., 'Consumer Satisfaction with Inpatient Psychiatric Treatment among Persons with Severe Mental Illness,' *Community Mental Health Journal* 43(6) (2006): 551–64.

50 See Richard Laugharne and Stefan Priebe, 'Trust, Choice, and Power in Mental Health: A Literature Review,' *Social Psychiatry and Psychiatric Epidemiology* 41(11) (2006): 843–52.

51 For example, Tom Burns et al., 'Treatment Challenges in Schizophrenia,' *Primary Care Psychiatry* 5(3) (1999): 117–23; Susan V. Eisen, Barbara Dickey, and Lloyd I. Sederer, 'A Self-Report Symptom and Problem Rating Scale to Increase Inpatients' Involvement in Treatment,' *Psychiatric Services* 51(3) (2000): 349–53.

52 Robert A. Clafferty, Elaine McCabe, and Keith W. Brown, 'Conspiracy of Silence? Telling Patients with Schizophrenia Their Diagnosis,' *Psychiatric Bulletin* 25(9) (2001): 336–9.

53 J.C. Day, P. Kinderman, and R. Bentall, 'A Comparison of Patients' and Prescribers' Beliefs about Neuroleptic Side Effects: Prevalence, Distress and Causation,' *Acta Psychiatrica Scandinavica* 97(1) (1998): 93–7.

54 It is very hard to determine exactly how many homeless people have a mental illness. Estimates vary widely and the proportion may change over time (see Sam Tsemberis and Rhonda F. Eisenberg, 'Pathways to Housing: Supported Housing for Street-Dwelling Homeless Individuals with Psychiatric Disabilities, *Psychiatric Services* 51 [2000]: 487–93; James C. Frankish et al., 'Homelessness and Health in Canada: Research Lessons and Priorities,' *Canadian Journal of Public Health* 96 [2005]: s23-s29; Carol S. North et al., 'Are Rates of Psychiatric Disorders in the Homeless Population Changing?' *American Journal of Public Health* 94(1) [2004]: 103–8). Perhaps more relevant to our research is a study (David Folsom et al., 'Prevalence and Risk Factors for Homelessness and Utilization of Mental Health Services among 10,340 Patients with Serious Mental Illness in a Large Public Mental Health System,' *American Journal of Psychiatry* 162(2) [2005]: 370–6) that found that 20 per cent of approximately five thousand people treated for schizophrenia were homeless at some point during the year of the study. This accords with the general feeling of the research group members that, based on their own experiences and the experiences of their colleagues, many people diagnosed with schizophrenia have difficulty finding and keeping stable housing.

55 For example, Stephan M. Goldfinger et al., 'Housing Placement and Sub-

sequent Days Homeless among Formerly Homeless Adults with Mental
Illness,' *Psychiatric Services* 50 (1999): 674–9; Patricia Hanrahan et al.,
'Housing Satisfaction and Service Use by Mentally Ill Persons in Community Integrated Living Arrangements,' *Psychiatric Services* 52 (2004):
1206–9; Frank R. Lipton, 'Tenure in Supportive Housing for Homeless
Persons with Severe Mental Illness,' *Psychiatric Services* 51 (2000): 479–486;
Frank R. Lipton, Suzanne Nutt, and Albert Sabitini, 'Housing the Home-
less Mentally Ill: A Longitudinal Study of a Treatment Approach,' *Hospital
and Community Psychiatry* 39 (1988): 40–5; David L. Shern et al., 'Hous-
ing Outcomes for Homeless Adults with Mental Illness: Results from the
Second-Round McKinney Program,' *Psychiatric Services* 48 (1997): 239–41;
Sam Tsemberis, Leyla Gulcur, and Maria Nakae, 'Housing First, Consumer Choice, and Harm Reduction for Homeless Individuals with a Dual
Diagnosis,' *American Journal of Public Health* 94(4) (2004): 651–6; Deborah
K. Padgett, Leyla Gulcur, and Sam Tsemberis, 'Housing First Services for
People Who Are Homeless with Co-Occurring Serious Mental Illness and
Substance Abuse,' *Research on Social Work Practice* 16(1) (2007): 74–83.
56 Lipton et al., 'Housing the Homeless.'
57 Tsemberis and Eisenberg, 'Pathways to Housing.'
58 Lipton et al., 'Housing the Homeless'; Tsemberis and Eisenberg, 'Pathways
to Housing.'
59 For example, Tsemberis et al., 'Housing First'; Tsembersi and Eisenberg,
'Pathways to Housing'; Padgett et al., 'Housing First Services'; Sam
Tsemberis, 'From Streets to Homes: An Innovative Approach to Supported
Housing from Homeless Adults with Psychiatric Disabilities,' *Journal of
Community Psychology* 27 (1999): 225–41; Ronni M. Greenwood et al., 'Decreasing Psychiatric Symptoms by Increasing Choice in Services for Adults
with Histories of Homelessness,' *American Journal of Community Psychol-
ogy* 36(3–4) (2005): 223–8; Leyla Gulcur et al., 'Housing, Hospitalization,
and Cost Outcomes for Homeless Individuals with Psychiatric Disabilities
Participating in Continuum or Care and Housing First Programmes,'
Journal of Community and Applied Social Psychology 13 (2003): 171–86; Philip
T. Yanos, S.M. Barrow, and Sam Tsemberis, 'Community Integration in the
Early Phase of Housing among Homeless Persons Diagnosed with Severe
Mental Illness: Successes and Challenges,' *Community Mental Health Journal*
40 (2004): 133–50; Sam Tsemberis et al., 'Consumer Preference Programs
for Individuals Who Are Homeless and Have Psychiatric Disabilities: A
Drop-In Center and a Supported Housing Program,' *American Journal of
Community Psychology* 32 (2003): 305–17.
60 Yanos et al., 'Community Integration.'

61 Colleen Clark and Alexander R. Rich, 'Outcomes of Homeless Adults in a Housing Program and in Case Management Only,' *Psychiatric Services* 54 (2003): 78–83.

62 Lipton et al., 'Tenure in Supportive Housing.'

63 See, for example, Beth Tanzman, 'An Overview of Surveys of Mental Health Consumers' Preferences of Housing and Support Services,' *Hospital and Community Psychiatry* 44 (1993): 450–5; D. Srebnik, J. Livingston, and L. Gordon, 'Housing Choice and Community Success for Individuals with Serious and Persistent Mental Illness,' *Community Mental Health Journal* 31 (1995): 139–52; R.K. Schutt and Stephan M. Goldfinger, 'Housing Preferences and Perceptions of Health and Functioning among Homeless Mentally Ill Persons,' *Psychiatric Services* 47 (1996): 381–6.

2: What We Did

1 Peter Beresford, 'A Service-User Perspective on Evidence,' in *Choosing Methods in Mental Health Research: Mental Health Research from Theory to Practice*, ed. Mike Slade and Stephen Priebe (New York: Routledge, 2006).

2 For example, Davidson et al., 'Purposes and Goals of Service User Involvement in Mental Health Research,' in *Handbook of Service User Involvement in Mental Health Research*, ed. Jan Wallcraft, Beate Schrank, and Michael Amering (London: Wiley, 2009); Peter Beresford, 'Theory and Practice of User Involvement in Research: Making the Connection with Public Policy and Practice,' in *Involving Service Users in Health and Social Care Research*, ed. Lesley Lowes and Ian Hulatt (London: Routledge, 2005), 6–17; Jonathan Boote, Rosemary Telford, and Cindy Cooper, 'Consumer Involvement in Health Research: A Review and Research Agenda,' *Health Policy* 61 (2002): 213–36.

3 See for example, Rose, 'Collaborative'; Alison Faulkner, 'Guidance for Good Practice,' SURGE UK Mental Health Research Network, http://www.mhrn.info/dnn/; Brenda Happell and Cath Roper, 'Consumer Participation in Mental Health Research: Articulating a Model to Guide Practice,' *Australian Psychiatry* 15(3) (2007): 237–41.

4 See Walsh and Boyle, 'Improving,' for an example of this kind of research.

5 See Joanna Ochocka, Rich Janzen, and Geoffrey Nelson, 'Sharing Power and Knowledge: Professional and Mental Health Consumer/Survivor Researchers Working Together in a Participatory Action Research Project,' *Psychiatric Rehabilitation Journal* 25(4) (2002): 379–87.

6 As a result of this meeting, Laurie, her therapist, Chris Austin, and I began a project in which Laurie and Chris wrote to each other as part of their

therapeutic interaction. Their experience of using writing as an aspect of therapy is published in Barbara Schneider, Chistopher Austin, and Laurie Arney, 'Writing to Wellness: Using Writing in Narrative Therapy,' *Journal of Systemic Therapies* 27(2) (2008): 42–57.

7 See, for example, Meredith Minkler and Nina Wallerstein, *Community-Based Participatory Research for Health* (San Francisco: Jossey-Bass, 2003).

3: What We Learned: Communication

1 Deegan, 'Recovery.'
2 Fisher, 'The Narrative Paradigm: An Elaboration,' *Communications Monographs* 52 (1985): 352.
3 Fisher, 'The Narrative Paradigm,' 353.

4: What We Learned: Housing

1 Nick Fox, 'Postmodern Perspectives on Care: The Vigil and the Gift,' *Critical Social Policy* 15 (44/45) (1995): 107–25.
2 Many scholars go further and identify control as an explicit goal of care. Irene Glasser and Rae Bridgeman (*Braving the Street: The Anthropology of Homelessness* [New York: Berghahn Books, 1999]) point out that 'charity has always underlined the differences between giver and receiver, and serves as a powerful element of social control' (40). Vincent Lyon-Callo (*Inequality, Poverty, and Neoliberal Governance: Activist Ethnography in the Homeless Sheltering Industry* [Peterborough: Broadview Press, 2004]) and Francis F. Piven and Richard A. Cloward (*Regulating the Poor: The Functions of Public Welfare* [New York: Pantheon, 1971]) identify social control of the poor as a goal of social welfare programs. Tom Allen (*Someone to Talk To: Care and Control of the Homeless* [Halifax: Fernwood, 2000]) describes social welfare as on the one hand being about helping people who are unable to 'keep up' and on the other hand as being about 'the regulation of people regarded as deficient' (12).
3 Fox 'Postmodern Perspectives,' 111.
4 Fox, 'Postmodern Perspectives,' 112.
5 Fox, 'Postmodern Perspectives,' 118.
6 Fox, 'Postmodern Perspectives,' 109.
7 Fox, 'Postmodern Perspectives,' 117.

5: Our Photovoice Project

1 CUPS Community Health Centre, *Calgary Street Talk*. Calgary: Calgary Ur-

ban Project Society (CUPS), http://www.cupshealthcentre.com/streettalk
.htm

2 Numerous websites offer information about photovoice. See, for example,
www.photovoice.ca.

3 Carolyn C. Wang, 'Using Photovoice as a Participatory Assessment and Issue Selection Tool,' in *Community Based Participatory Research for Heath*, ed.
Meredith Minkler and Nina Wallerstein (San Francisco: Jossey-Bass, 2003),
179.

4 Carolyn C. Wang, 'Photovoice: A Participatory Action Research Strategy
Applied to Women's Health,' *Journal of Women's Health* 8(2) (1999): 185.

5 Carolyn C. Wang and Mary Ann Burris, 'Empowerment through Photo
Novellas: Portraits of Participation,' *Health Education Quarterly* 21(2) (1994):
171–86. Carolyn C. Wang, and Mary Ann Burris, 'Photovoice: Concept,
Methodology, and Use for Participatory Needs Assessment,' *Health, Education and Behavior* 24(3) (1997): 369–87; Carolyn C. Wang et al., 'Photovoice
as a Participatory Health Promotion Strategy,' *Health Promotion International* 13(1) (1998): 775–86.

6 Photovoice projects have been carried out in a variety of topic areas and
disciplines. They have highlighted the experiences of mothers with learning disabilities and their children (Tim Booth and Wendy Booth, 'In the
Frame: Photo Voice and Mothers with Learning Difficulties,' *Disability
and Society* 18(4) [2003]: 431–42); explored the care needs of the elderly
after they have been discharged from hospital (Chantale M. LeClerc et al.,
'Falling Short of the Mark: Tales of Life after Hospital Discharge,' *Clinical
Nursing Research* 11(3) [2002]: 242–63); and investigated educational development among health care professionals (Robin G. Riley and Elizabeth
Manias, 'The Uses of Photography in Clinical Nursing Practice and Research: A Literature Review,' *Journal of Advanced Nursing* 48(4) [2004]: 397–
405; Carolyn C. Wang, Robert M. Anderson, and David T. Stern, 'Exploring
Professional Values and Health Policy through Photovoice,' *Medical Education* 38 [2004]: 1190–1; Fern W. Goodhart et al., 'A View through a Different
Lens: Photovoice as a Tool for Student Advocacy,' *Journal of American College Health* 55[July/August 2006]: 53–6). The ease with which participants
can document their experiences makes it a useful approach for people
who have severe health challenges such as chronic pain (Tamara A. Baker
and Carolyn Wang, 'Photovoice: Use of a Participatory Action Research
Method to Explore the Chronic Pain Experience in Older Adults,' *Qualitative Health Research* 16(10) [2006]: 1405–13). In Calgary, photovoice has been
used to illustrate the experiences of women who live in poverty and struggle to find fair wage employment (Lynda Laughlin, Donna McPhee, and
Maggie Pompeo, 'Women's Perspectives on Poverty: Photos and Stories by

Women on Low-Income in Calgary' [Calgary: Women and a Fair Income Project, 2004]). http://www.ucalgary.ca/gender/files/WAFI%20Report2 .pdf) (accessed 20 November 2009).

7 John Gaventa, 'The Powerful, the Powerless, and the Experts: Knowledge Struggles in an Information Age,' in *Voices of Change: Participatory Research in the United States and Canada*, ed. Peter Park, Mary Brydon-Miller, Budd Hall, and Ted Jackson (Toronto: Ontario Institute for Studies in Education, 1993), 40.

8 Alan Radley, Darrin Hodgetts, and Andrea Cullen, 'Visualizing Homelessness: A Study in Photography and Estrangement,' *Journal of Community and Applied Social Psychology* 15 (2005): 273–95.

9 Carolyn C. Wang, Jennifer L. Cash, and Lisa S. Powers, 'Who Knows the Streets as Well as the Homeless? Promoting Personal and Community Action through Photovoice,' *Health Promotion Practice* 1(1) (2000): 81–9.

10 Christine Walsh, Gayle Rutherford, and Larissa Muller, *Home: Perspectives of Women Who Are Homeless* (Calgary: University of Calgary, 2007).

11 M. Dixon and M. Hadjialexiou, 'Photovoice: Promising Practice in Engaging Young People Who Are Homeless,' *Youth Studies Australia* 24(2) (2005): 52–6.

12 Carolyn C. Wang and Cheri A. Pies, 'Family, Maternal, and Child Health through Photovoice,' *Maternal and Child Care* 8(2) (2004): 95–102.

6: Taking Action

1 Daryl Rock, 'Knowledge Mobilization and the Consumer: "Whatever Happened to the Research You Funded?"' *Abilities* 59 (2004): 32.

2 Ross E. Gray and Christina Sinding, *Standing Ovation: Performing Social Science Research about Cancer* (Walnut Creek: Altamira, 2002); Ross E. Gray, Vrenia Ivonoffski, and Christina Sinding, 'Making a Mess and Spreading It Around: Articulation of an Approach to Research-Based Theatre,' in *Ethnographically Speaking: Autoethnography, Literature, and Aesthetics*, ed. Arthur P. Bochner and Carolyn Ellis (New York: Rowman and Littlefield, 2001), 57–75.

3 A number of fascinating examples exist of the use of theatre to disseminate research. Jim Mienczakowski ('Ethnodrama: Performed Research – Limitations and Potential,' in *Handbook of Ethnography*, ed. Paul Atkinson, Amanda Coffey, Sara Delamont, et al. [London: Sage, 2001], 468–76, and 'The Theatre of Ethnography: The Reconstruction of Ethnography into Theatre with Emancipatory Potential,' *Qualitative Inquiry* 1 [1995]: 360–75) has produced performances about the health care experiences of people di-

agnosed with schizophrenia and about the experiences of people in a drug and alcohol detox centre. Joan M. Eakin and Marion Endicott ('Knowledge Translation through Research-Based Theatre,' *Healthcare Policy* 2(2) [2006]: 54–9) used theatre to disseminate results from their study of Ontario's system for reducing disability from work-related injury. Della Pollock ('Telling the Story: Performing Like a Family,' *Oral History Review* 18 [1990]: 1–36) produced a play based on three hundred interviews with former cotton mill workers in South Carolina. Marianne A. Paget ('Performing the Text,' *Journal of Contemporary Ethnography* 19 [1990]: 136–55) dramatized the interaction of doctor and patient in the case of a woman being diagnosed with cancer. Harold S. Becker and his colleagues ('Theatres and Communities: Three Scenes,' *Social Problems* 36 [1989]: 93–116) created a performance based on interviews with theatre directors, actors, and other theatre workers in three metropolitan areas in the US.

4 Norman K. Denzin, 'The Many Faces of Emotionality,' in *Investigating Subjectivity: Research on Lived Experience*, ed. Carolyn Ellis (London: Sage, 1992), 20.

5 Andrew Sparkes, 'Autoethnography and Narratives of Self: Reflections on Criteria in Action,' *Sociology of Sport Journal* 17 (2000): 22.

6 For example, Ellis and Bochner, 'Autoethnography'; Paget, 'Performing'; Becker et al., 'Theatres and Communities'; Sparkes, 'Autoethnography'; Bochner and Ellis, *Ethnographically Speaking*; Dwight Conquergood, 'Rethinking Ethnography: Towards a Critical Cultural Politics,' *Communication Monographs* 58 (1991): 179–94.

7 Denzin, *Performance Ethnography*; Laurel Richardson, 'Poetic Representation of Interviews,' in *Handbook of Interview Research*, ed. Jaber F. Gubrium and James A. Holstein (Thousand Oaks: Sage, 2002), 923–48.

8 Mary M. Gergen and Kenneth J. Gergen, 'Ethnographic Presentation as Relationship,' in *Ethnographically Speaking: Autoethnography, Literature, and Aesthetics*, ed. Arthur P. Bochner and Carolyn Ellis (New York: Rowman and Littlefield, 2001), 19.

9 Gergen and Gergen, 'Ethnographic Presentation,' 31.

10 Gergen and Gergen, 'Ethnographic Presentation,' 12.

11 Gergen and Gergen, 'Ethnographic Presentation,' 19.

12 Lauren Berger, 'Inside Out: Narrative Auto Ethnography as a Path toward Rapport,' *Qualitative Inquiry* 7 (2001): 508.

13 Ursula Franklin, *The Ursula Franklin Reader: Pacifism as a Map* (Toronto: Between the Lines, 2006).

14 See for example http://www.aaronshep.com/rt/.

15 See for example http://en.wikipedia.org/wiki/Citizen media.

7: Where We Got To

1 Alison Faulkner, *The Ethics of Survivor Research: Guidelines for the Ethical Conduct of Research Carried Out by Mental Health Service Users and Survivors* (Bristol, UK: Polity Press, 2004); Beresford, 'Theory and Practice.' See also Wallcraft et al., *Handbook*.

Epilogue

1 Davidson, *Living outside Mental Illness*, 1. For an example of qualitative mental health housing research see Geoffrey Nelson et al., 'A Narrative Approach to the Evaluation of Supported Housing: Stories of Homeless People Who Have Experienced Serious Mental Illness,' *Psychiatric Rehabilitation Journal* 29(2) (2004): 98–104.
2 See Ruth Lister, 'Inclusive Citizenship: Realizing the Potential,' *Citizenship Studies* 11(1) (2007): 49–61; Naila Kabeer, *Inclusive Citizenship: Meanings and Expressions* (London and New York: Zed Books, 2005); Jenny Morris, *Citizenship and Disability* (London: Disability Rights Commission, 2005). Citizenship is a highly contested term with many uses and meanings. We use the term in the way that scholars interested in inclusive citizenship do, with a focus on recognition and membership rather than on the traditional areas of formal rights or the relationship between the individual and the state. Full citizenship in this view offers recognition of difference and a right to full cultural participation.

References

Alexander, Bryant K. 'Performance Ethnography: The Reenacting and Inciting of Culture.' In *The Sage Handbook of Qualitative Research*, 3rd edition, edited by Norman K. Denzin and Yvonna S. Lincoln, 411–42. Thousand Oaks: Sage, 2005.

Allen, Tom. *Someone to Talk To: Care and Control of the Homeless*. Halifax: Fernwood, 2000.

Andreason, Nancy. *The Broken Brain: The Biological Revolution in Psychiatry*. New York: Harper and Row, 1984.

Baker, Tamara A., and Carolyn Wang. 'Photovoice: Use of a Participatory Action Research Method to Explore the Chronic Pain Experience in Older Adults.' *Qualitative Health Research* 16(10) (2006): 1405–13.

Balcazar, Fabricio, Christopher B. Keys, Daniel L. Kaplan, and Yolande Suarez-Balcazar. 'Participatory Research and People with Disabilities: Principles and Challenges.' *Canadian Journal of Rehabilitation* 12 (1999): 105–12.

Becker, Harold S., Michael M. McCall, L.V. Morris, and P. Meshijan. 'Theatres and Communities: Three Scenes.' *Social Problems* 36 (1989): 93–116.

Beresford, Peter. 'Theory and Practice of User Involvement in Research: Making the Connection with Public Policy and Practice.' In *Involving Service Users in Health and Social Care Research*, edited by Lesley Lowes and Ian Hulatt, 6–17. London: Routledge, 2005.

– 'A Service-User Perspective on Evidence.' In *Choosing Methods in Mental Health Research: Mental Health Research from Theory to Practice*, edited by Mike Slade and Stephen Priebe, 223–30. New York: Routledge, 2006.

Berger, Lauren. 'Inside Out: Narrative Auto Ethnography as a Path toward Rapport.' *Qualitative Inquiry* 7 (2001): 504–18.

Bochner, Arthur P., and Carolyn E. Ellis, eds. *Ethnographically Speaking: Autoethnography, Literature, and Aesthetics*. New York: Rowman and Littlefield, 2001.

Boote, Jonathan, Rosemary Telford, and Cindy Cooper. 'Consumer Involvement in Health Research: A Review and Research Agenda.' *Health Policy* 61 (2002): 213–36.

Booth, Tim, and Wendy Booth. 'In the Frame: Photo Voice and Mothers with Learning Difficulties.' *Disability and Society* 18(4) (2003): 431–42.

Burns, Tom, D. Baldwin, R. Emsley, R. Kerwin, J. Steinberg, and J. Van Os. 'Treatment Challenges in Schizophrenia.' *Primary Care Psychiatry* 5(3) (1999): 117–23.

Calgary Homeless Foundation. *Calgary Community Plan: Building Paths out of Homelessness.* Calgary: Calgary Homeless Foundation, 2003.

Campbell, Jean, and R. Schreiber. *In Pursuit of Wellness: The Well-Being Project.* Sacramento: California Department of Mental Health, 1989.

Canadian Nurses Association. *Preparation for Community Living: The Bridge to Discharge Project.* Ottawa: Canadian Nurses Association, 1996.

Chaney, RoAnne. 'The Value of Consumer Involvement in Medicaid Managed Care.' Centre for Health Care Strategies Brief. http://www.chcs.org/usr_doc/consumer_involvement.pdf (accessed 21 January 2008).

Ciompi, Luc. 'Catamnestic Long-Term Study on the Course of Life and Aging of Schizophrenics.' *Schizophrenia Bulletin* 6 (1980): 606–18.

Ciompi, Luc. 'The Natural History of Schizophrenia in the Long Term.' *British Journal of Psychiatry* 136 (1980): 413–20.

Clafferty, Robert. A., Elaine McCabe, and Keith W. Brown. 'Conspiracy of Silence? Telling Patients with Schizophrenia Their Diagnosis.' *Psychiatric Bulletin* 25(9) (2001): 336–9.

Clark, Colleen, and Alexander R. Rich. 'Outcomes of Homeless Adults in a Housing Program and in Case Management Only.' *Psychiatric Services* 54 (2003): 78–83.

Conquergood, Dwight. 'Rethinking Ethnography: Towards a Critical Cultural Politics.' *Communication Monographs* 58 (1991): 179–94.

CUPS Community Health Centre. *Calgary Street Talk.* Calgary: Calgary Urban Project Society (CUPS), http://www.cupshealthcentre.com/streettalk.htm

Davidson, Larry. *Living outside Mental Illness: Qualitative Studies of Recovery in Schizophrenia.* New York: New York University Press, 2003.

Davidson, Larry, and Thomas H. McGlashan. 'The Varied Outcomes of Schizophrenia.' *Canadian Journal of Psychiatry* 42(1) (1997): 34–43.

Davidson, Larry, Patricia Ridgway, Timothy Schmutte, and Maria O'Connell. 'Purposes and Goals of Service User Involvement in Mental Health Research.' In *Handbook of Service User Involvement in Mental Health Research,* edited by Jan Wallcraft, Beate Schrank, and Michael Amering. London: Wiley, 2009.

Davidson, Larry, David A. Stayner, Stacey Lambert, Peter Smith, and William H. Sledge. 'Phenomenological and Participatory Research on Schizophrenia: Recovering the Person in Theory and Practice.' In *From Subjects to Subjectivities: A Handbook of Interpretive and Participatory Methods*, edited by Deborah L. Tolman and Mary Brydon-Miller, 163–79. New York: New York University Press, 2001.

Day, J.C., P. Kinderman, and R. Bentall. ' A Comparison of Patients' and Prescribers' Beliefs about Neuroleptic Side Effects: Prevalence, Distress and Causation.' *Acta Psychiatrica Scandinavica* 97(1) (1998): 93–7.

Deegan, Patricia. 'Recovery: The Lived Experience of Rehabilitation.' *Psychosocial Rehabilitation Journal* 15(3) (1988): 3–19.

Delman, Jonathan. 'Consumer-Driven and Conducted Survey Research in Action.' In *Towards Best Practices for Surveying People with Disabilities*, edited by Thilo Kroll, Juliana Cyril, Paul O. Placek, and Gerry Hendershot, 71–87. Hauppage, NY: Nova Science, 2007.

Denzin, Norman K. 'The Many Faces of Emotionality.' In *Investigating Subjectivity: Research on Lived Experience*, edited by Carolyn Ellis, 17–30. London: Sage, 1992.

– *Interpretive Ethnography: Ethnographic Practices for the 21st Century.* Thousand Oaks: Sage, 1997.

– *Performance Ethnography: Critical Pedagogy and the Politics of Culture.* Thousand Oaks: Sage, 2003.

Dixon, M., and M. Hadjialexiou. 'Photovoice: Promising Practice in Engaging Young People Who Are Homeless.' *Youth Studies Australia* 24(2) (2005): 52–6.

Eakin, Joan M., and Marion Endicott. 'Knowledge Translation through Research-Based Theatre.' *Healthcare Policy* 2(2) (2006): 54–9.

Eisen, Susan V., Barbara Dickey, and Lloyd I. Sederer. 'A Self-Report Symptom and Problem Rating Scale to Increase Inpatients' Involvement in Treatment.' *Psychiatric Services* 51(3) (2000): 349–53.

Ellis, Carolyn, and Arthur P. Bochner. 'Autoethnography, Personal Narrative, Reflexivity: Researcher as Subject.' In *Handbook of Qualitative Research*, 2nd edition, edited by Norman K. Denzin and Yvonna S. Lincoln, 733–68. Thousand Oaks: Sage, 2000.

Fals-Borda, Orlando, and Muhammad Anisur Rahman, eds. *Action and Knowledge: Breaking the Monopoly with Participatory Action Research.* New York: Intermediate Technology/Apex, 1991.

Faulkner, Alison. *The Ethics of Survivor Research: Guidelines for the Ethical Conduct of Research Carried Out by Mental Health Service Users and Survivors.* Bristol, UK: Polity Press, 2004.

– 'Guidance for Good Practice.' SURGE UK Mental Health Research Network, n.d.. http://www.mhrn.info/dnn/ (accessed 26 April 2008).

Faulkner, Alison, and Sarah Layzell. *Strategies for Living: A Report of User-Led Research into People's Strategies for Living with Mental Distress.* London: Mental Health Foundation, 2001.

Faulkner, Alison, and Phil Thomas. 'User-Led Research and Evidence-Based Medicine.' *British Journal of Psychiatry* 180(1) (2002): 1–3.

Fisher, Walter R. 'Narration as a Human Communication Paradigm.' *Communication Monographs* 51 (1984): 1–22.

– 'The Narrative Paradigm: An Elaboration.' *Communication Monographs* 52 (1985): 347–67.

– *Human Communication as Narration: Towards a Philosophy of Reason, Value, and Action.* Columbia: University of South Carolina Press, 1987.

– 'Narration, Reason, and Community.' In *Memory, Identity, Community: The Idea of Narrative in the Human Sciences,* edited by L.P. Hinchman and S.K. Hinchman, 307–27. Albany: State University of New York Press, 1997.

Folsom, David, W. Hawthorne, L. Lindamer, T. Gilmer, A. Bailey, S. Golshan, P. Garcia, J. Unützer, R. Hough, and D. Juste. 'Prevalence and Risk Factors for Homelessness and Utilization of Mental Health Services among 10,340 Patients with Serious Mental Illness in a Large Public Mental Health System.' *American Journal of Psychiatry* 162(2) (2005): 370–6.

Forchuk, Cheryl, J. Jewell, R. Schofield, M. Sircelj, and T. Valledor. 'From Hospital to Community: Bridging Therapeutic Relationships.' *Journal of Psychiatric and Mental Health Nursing* 5 (1998): 197–202.

Fox, Nick. 'Postmodern Perspectives on Care: The Vigil and the Gift.' *Critical Social Policy* 15 (44/55) (1995): 107–25.

Frankish, James C., Stephen W. Hwang, and Darryl Quant. 'Homelessness and Health in Canada: Research Lessons and Priorities.' *Canadian Journal of Public Health* 96 (2005): s23-s29.

Franklin, Ursula. *The Ursula Franklin Reader: Pacifism as a Map.* Toronto: Between the Lines, 2006.

Gaventa, John. 'The Powerful, the Powerless, and the Experts: Knowledge Struggles in an Information Age.' In *Voices of Change: Participatory Research in the United States and Canada,* edited by Peter Park, Mary Brydon-Miller, Budd Hall, and Ted Jackson. Toronto: Ontario Institute for Studies in Education, 1993.

Gergen, Mary M., and Kenneth J. Gergen. 'Ethnographic Presentation as Relationship.' In *Ethnographically Speaking: Autoethnography, Literature, and Aesthetics,* edited by Arthur P. Bochner and Carolyn Ellis, 11–33. New York: Rowman and Littlefield, 2001.

Glasser, Irene, and Rae Bridgeman. *Braving the Street: The Anthropology of Homelessness*. New York: Berghahn Books, 1999.

Goldfinger, Stephan M., R.K. Schutt, G.S. Tolomiczenko, L. Seidman, W.E. Penk, W. Turner, and B. Caplan. 'Housing Placement and Subsequent Days Homeless among Formerly Homeless Adults with Mental Illness.' *Psychiatric Services* 50 (1999): 674–9.

Goodhart, Fern W., J. Hsu, J.H. Baek, A.L. Coleman, F.M. Maresca, and M.B. Miller. 'A View through a Different Lens: Photovoice as a Tool for Student Advocacy.' *Journal of American College Health* 55 (July/August 2006): 53–6.

Gray, Ross E., Vrenia Ivonoffski, and Christina Sinding. 'Making a Mess and Spreading It Around: Articulation of an Approach to Research-Based Theatre.' In *Ethnographically Speaking: Autoethnography, Literature, and Aesthetics*, edited by Arthur P. Bochner and Carolyn Ellis, 57–75. New York: Rowman and Littlefield, 2001.

Gray, Ross E., and Christina Sinding. *Standing Ovation: Performing Social Science Research about Cancer*. Walnut Creek: Altamira, 2002.

Greene, Michael F. *Schizophrenia Revealed: From Neurons to Social Interactions*. New York: W.W. Norton and Company, 2001.

Greenwood, Ronni M, Nicole Schaefer-McDaniel, Gary Winkel, and Sam Tsemberis. 'Decreasing Psychiatric Symptoms by Increasing Choice in Services for Adults with Histories of Homelessness.' *American Journal of Community Psychology* 36(3–4) (2005): 223–38.

Gulcur, Leyla, Ana Stefanic, Marybeth Shinn, Sam Tsemberis, and Sean Fischer. 'Housing, Hospitalization, and Cost Outcomes for Homeless Individuals with Psychiatric Disabilities Participating in Continuum of Care and Housing First Programmes.' *Journal of Community and Applied Social Psychology* 13 (2003): 171–86.

Hackman, Anna, C. Brown, Y. Yang, R. Goldberg, J. Kreyenbuhl, A. Lucksted, K. Wohlheiter, and L. Dixon. 'Consumer Satisfaction with Inpatient Psychiatric Treatment among Persons with Severe Mental Illness.' *Community Mental Health Journal* 43(6) (2006): 551–64.

Hall, Budd. 'Introduction.' In *Voices of Change: Participatory Research in the United States and Canada*, edited by Peter Park, Mary Brydon-Miller, Budd Hall, and Ted Jackson, xiii–xxii. Toronto: OISE Press, 1993.

Hanrahan, Patricia, D.J. Luchins, C. Savage, and H. Goldman. 'Housing Satisfaction and Service Use by Mentally Ill Persons in Community Integrated Living Arrangements.' *Psychiatric Services* 52 (2004): 1206–9.

Happell, Brenda, and Cath Roper. 'Consumer Participation in Mental Health Research: Articulating a Model to Guide Practice.' *Australian Psychiatry* 15(3) (2007): 237–41.

Harding, Courtney M., G.W. Brooks, T. Ashikaga, J.S. Strauss, and A. Breier. 'The Vermont Longitudinal Study of Persons with Severe Mental Illness, I: Methodology, Study Sample, and Overall Status 32 Years Later.' *American Journal of Psychiatry* 144(6) (1987a): 718–26.

Harding, Courtney M., G.W. Brooks, T. Ashikaga, J.S. Strauss, and A. Breier. 'The Longitudinal Study of Persons with Severe Mental Illness, II: Long-Term Outcome of Subjects Who Retrospectively Met DSMIII Criteria for Schizophrenia.' *American Journal of Psychiatry* 144(6) (1987b): 727–35.

Harding, Courtney M., and James H. Zahniser. 'Empirical Correction of Seven Myths about Schizophrenia with Implications for Treatment.' *Acta Psychiatrica Scandinavica* 90 (supp. 384) (1994): 140–6.

Hornung, W.P., S. Klingberg, R. Feldmann, K. Schonauer, and H. Schulze Monking. 'Collaboration with Drug Treatment by Schizophrenic Patients with and without Psychoeducational Training: Results of a One-Year Followup.' *Acta Psychiatrica Scandinavica* 97(3) (1998): 213–19.

Jacobson, Nora, and Dianne Greenley. 'What Is Recovery? A Conceptual Model and Explanation.' *Psychiatric Services* 52(4) (2001): 482–5.

Kabeer, Naila. *Inclusive Citizenship: Meanings and Expressions.* London and New York: Zed Books, 2005.

Kemmis, Stephen, and Robin McTaggart. 'Participatory Action Research: Communicative Action and the Public Sphere.' In *Handbook of Qualitative Research*, 3rd edition, edited by Norman K. Denzin and Yvonna S. Lincoln, 559–604. Newbury Park: Sage, 2005.

Laing, R.D. *The Politics of Experience.* New York: Pantheon, 1967.

Laugharne, Richard, and Stephan Priebe. 'Trust, Choice, and Power in Mental Health: A Literature Review.' *Social Psychiatry and Psychiatric Epidemiology* 41(11) (2006): 843–52.

Laughlin, Lynda, Donna McPhee, and Maggie Pompeo. 'Women's Perspectives on Poverty: Photos and Stories by Women on Low-Income in Calgary.' Calgary: Women and a Fair Income Project, 2004. http://www.ucalgary.ca/gender/files/WAFI%20Report2.pdf (accessed 14 April 2008).

LeClerc, Chantale M., D.L. Wells, D. Craig, and J.L. Wilson. 'Falling Short of the Mark: Tales of Life after Hospital Discharge.' *Clinical Nursing Research* 11(3) (2002): 242–63.

Lipton, Frank R., Suzanne Nutt, and Albert Sabitini. 'Housing the Homeless Mentally Ill: A Longitudinal Study of a Treatment Approach.' *Hospital and Community Psychiatry* 39 (1988): 40–5.

Lipton, Frank R., C. Siegel, A. Hannigan, J. Samuels, and S. Baker. 'Tenure in Supportive Housing for Homeless Persons with Severe Mental Illness.' *Psychiatric Services* 51 (2000): 479–86.

Lister, Ruth. 'Inclusive Citizenship: Realizing the Potential.' *Citizenship Studies* 11(1) (2007): 49–61.

Llewellyn-Jones, Sian, Gill Jones, and Peter Donnely. 'Questions Patients Ask Psychiatrists.' *Psychiatric Bulletin* 25(1) (2001): 21–4.

Lyon-Callo, Vincent. *Inequality, Poverty, and Neoliberal Governance: Activist Ethnography in the Homeless Sheltering Industry.* Peterborough: Broadview Press, 2004.

Manitoba Schizophrenia Society. *The Truth about Schizophrenia: Why You Should Change Your Thinking about Youth's Greatest Disabler.* Winnipeg: Manitoba Schizophrenia Society, 2000.

McGuire, Patrick A. 'New Hope for People with Schizophrenia.' *Monitor on Psychology* 31(2) (2000). http://www.apa.org/monitor/feb00/schizophrenia.html (accessed 21 January 2008).

McKnight, John L., and John P. Kretzmann. 'Mapping Community Capacity.' In *Community Organizing and Community Building for Health,* edited by Meredith Minkler, 158–72. New Brunswick: Rutgers University Press, 2006.

Mienczakowski, Jim. 'The Theatre of Ethnography: The Reconstruction of Ethnography into Theatre with Emancipatory Potential.' *Qualitative Inquiry* 1 (1995): 360–75.

– 'Ethnodrama: Performed Research – Limitations and Potential.' In *Handbook of Ethnography,* edited by Paul Atkinson, Amanda Coffey, Sarah Delamont, John Lofland, and Lyn Lofland, 468–76. London: Sage, 2001.

Minkler, Meredith, and Nina Wallerstein. *Community-Based Participatory Research for Health.* San Francisco: Jossey-Bass, 2003.

Morris, Jenny. *Citizenship and Disability.* London: Disability Rights Commission, 2005. http://www.leeds.ac.uk/disability-studies/archiveuk/morris/Citizenship (accessed 18 May 2008).

Morrison, Linda. *Talking Back to Psychiatry: The Psychiatric Consumer/Survivor/Ex-Patient Movement.* New York: Routledge, 2005.

Nelson, Geoffrey, Juanne Clarke, Angela Febbraro, and Maria Hatzipantelis. 'A Narrative Approach to the Evaluation of Supported Housing: Stories of Homeless People Who Have Experienced Serious Mental Illness.' *Psychiatric Rehabilitation Journal* 29(2) (2004): 98–104.

North, Carol S., K.M. Eyrich, D.E. Pollio, and E.L. Spitznagel. 'Are Rates of Psychiatric Disorders in the Homeless Population Changing?' *American Journal of Public Health* 94(1) (2004): 103–8.

Ochocka, Joanna, Rich Janzen, and Geoffrey Nelson. 'Sharing Power and Knowledge: Professional and Mental Health Consumer/Survivor Researchers Working Together in a Participatory Action Research Project.' *Psychiatric Rehabilitation Journal* 25(4) (2002): 379–87.

Oehl, M., M. Hummer, and W.W. Fleischhacker. 'Compliance with Antipsychotic Treatment.' *Acta Psychiatrica Scandinavica* 102(6) (2000): 83–7.

Oliver, Michael. 'Changing the Social Relations of Research Production?' *Disability, Handicap, and Society* 7 (1992): 101–14.

Padgett, Deborah K., Leyla Gulcur, and Sam Tsemberis. 'Housing First Services for People Who Are Homeless with Co-Occurring Serious Mental Illness and Substance Abuse.' *Research on Social Work Practice* 16(1) (2007): 74–83.

Paget, Marianne A. 'Performing the Text.' *Journal of Contemporary Ethnography* 19 (1990): 136–55.

Pilgrim, David. *Key Concepts in Mental Health*. London: Sage, 2005.

Piven, Francis F., and Richard A. Cloward. *Regulating the Poor: The Functions of Public Welfare*. New York: Pantheon, 1971.

Pollock, Della. 'Telling the Story: Performing Like a Family.' *Oral History Review* 18 (1990): 1–36.

Radley, Alan, Darrin Hodgetts, and Andrea Cullen. 'Visualizing Homelessness: A Study in Photography and Estrangement.' *Journal of Community and Applied Social Psychology* 15 (2005): 273–95.

Reason, Peter. 'Three Approaches to Participative Inquiry.' In *Handbook of Qualitative Research*, 1st edition, edited by Norman K. Denzin and Yvonna S. Lincoln, 324–39. Newbury Park: Sage, 1994.

Reason, Peter, and Hilary Bradbury. 'Introduction: Inquiry and Participation in Search of a World Worthy of Human Aspiration.' In *Handbook of Action Research: The Concise Paperback Edition*, edited by Peter Reason and Hilary Bradbury, 1–14. London: Sage, 2006.

Richardson, Laurel. 'Poetic Representation of Interviews.' In *Handbook of Interview Research*, edited by Jaber F. Gubrium and James A. Holstein, 923–48. Thousand Oaks: Sage, 2002.

Riley, Robin G., and Elizabeth Manias. 'The Uses of Photography in Clinical Nursing Practice and Research: A Literature Review.' *Journal of Advanced Nursing* 48(4) (2004): 397–405.

Rock, Daryl. 'Knowledge Mobilization and the Consumer: "Whatever Happened to the Research You Funded?"' *Abilities* 59 (2004): 32.

Rose, Diana. *Users' Voices: The Perspectives of Mental Health Service Users on Community and Hospital Care*. London: Sainsbury Centre for Mental Health, 2001.

– 'Collaborative Research between Users and Professionals: Peaks and Pitfalls.' *Psychiatric Bulletin* 27 (2003): 404–6.

Schneider, Barbara. 'Narratives of Schizophrenia: Constructing a Positive Identity.' *Canadian Journal of Communication* 28(2) (2003): 185–201.

– 'Mothers Talk about Their Children with Schizophrenia: A Performance Authoethnography.' *Journal of Psychiatric and Mental Health Nursing* 12 (2005): 333–40.

Schneider, Barbara, Chistopher Austin, and Laurie Arney. 'Writing to Wellness: Using Writing in Narrative Therapy.' *Journal of Systemic Therapies* 27(2) (2008): 42–57.

Schneider, Barbara, Hannah Scissons, Laurie Arney, George Benson, Jeff Derry, Ken Lucas, Michele Misurelli, Dana Nickerson, and Mark Sunderland. 'Communication between People with Schizophrenia and Their Medical Professionals: A Participatory Research Project.' *Qualitative Health Research* 14 (2004): 562–77.

Schutt, R.K, and Stephan M. Goldfinger. 'Housing Preferences and Perceptions of Health and Functioning among Homeless Mentally Ill Persons.' *Psychiatric Services* 47 (1996): 381–6.

Shern, David L., C.J. Felton, R.L. Hough, A.F. Lehman, S. Goldfinger, D. Valencia, D. Dennis, R. Straw, and P.A. Wood. 'Housing Outcomes for Homeless Adults with Mental Illness: Results from the Second-Round McKinney Program.' *Psychiatric Services* 48 (1997): 239–41.

Sparkes, Andrew. 'Autoethnography and Narratives of Self: Reflections on Criteria in Action.' *Sociology of Sport Journal* 17 (2000): 21–43.

Spry, Tami. 'Performing Autoethnography: An Embodied Methodological Praxis.' *Qualitative Inquiry* 7 (2001): 706–32.

Srebnik, D., J. Livingston, and L. Gordon. 'Housing Choice and Community Success for Individuals with Serious and Persistent Mental Illness.' *Community Mental Health Journal* 31 (1995): 139–52.

Sweeney, Angela, Peter Beresford, Alison Faulkner, Mary Nettle, and Diana Rose, eds. *This Is Survivor Research.* Ross-on-Wye, UK: PCCS Books, 2009.

Szasz, Thomas. *The Myth of Mental Illness: Foundations of a Theory of Personal Conduct.* New York: Harper and Row, 1974.

Tanzman, Beth. 'An Overview of Surveys of Mental Health Consumers' Preferences of Housing and Support Services.' *Hospital and Community Psychiatry* 44 (1993): 450–5.

Thompson, Teresa L., Alice M. Dorsey, Katherine I. Miller, and Roxanne Parrot, eds. *Handbook of Health Communication.* London: Laurence Erlbaum Associates, 2003.

Torrey, E. Fuller. *Surviving Schizophrenia: A Manual for Families, Consumers, and Providers.* 5th edition. New York: HarperCollins, 2006.

Tsemberis, Sam. 'From Streets to Homes: An Innovative Approach to Supported Housing from Homeless Adults with Psychiatric Disabilities.' *Journal of Community Psychology* 27 (1999): 225–41.

Tsemberis, Sam, and Rhonda F. Eisenberg. 'Pathways to Housing: Supported Housing for Street-Dwelling Homeless Individuals with Psychiatric Disabilities.' *Psychiatric Services* 51 (2000): 487–93.

Tsemberis, Sam, Leyla Gulcur, and Maria Nakae. 'Housing First, Consumer Choice, and Harm Reduction for Homeless Individuals with a Dual Diagnosis.' *American Journal of Public Health* 94(4) (2004): 651–6.

Tsemberis, Sam, L. Moran, M. Shinn, S.M. Asmussen, and David L. Shern. 'Consumer Preference Programs for Individuals Who Are Homeless and Have Psychiatric Disabilities: A Drop-In Center and a Supported Housing Program.' *American Journal of Community Psychology* 32 (2003): 305–17.

Turner, Michael, and Peter Beresford. *User Controlled Research: Its Meanings and Potential. Final Report*. Brunel University: Shaping Our Lives and the Centre for Citizen Participation, 2005. http://www.invo.org.uk/Commissioned_Work.asp (accessed 16 March 2009).

Wallcraft, Jan, Beate Schrank, and Michael Amering, eds. *Handbook of Service User Involvement in Mental Health Research*. London: Wiley, 2009.

Walsh, Christine, Gayle Rutherford, and Larissa Muller. 'Home: Perspectives of Women Who Are Homeless.' Calgary: University of Calgary, 2007.

Walsh, Jim, and Joan Boyle. 'Improving Acute Psychiatric Hospital Services According to Inpatient Experiences: A User-Led Piece of Research as a Means to Empowerment.' *Issues in Mental Health Nursing* 30(1) (2009): 31–8.

Wang, Carolyn C. 'Photovoice: A Participatory Action Research Strategy Applied to Women's Health.' *Journal of Women's Health* 8(2) (1999): 185–92.

– 'Using Photovoice as a Participatory Assessment and Issue Selection Tool.' In *Community Based Participatory Research for Heath*, edited by Meredith Minkler and Nina Wallerstein, 179–86. San Francisco: Jossey-Bass, 2003.

Wang, Carolyn C., Robert M. Anderson, and David T. Stern. 'Exploring Professional Values and Health Policy through Photovoice.' *Medical Education* 38 (2004): 1190–1.

Wang, Carolyn C., and Mary Ann Burris. 'Empowerment through Photo Novellas: Portraits of Participation.' *Health Education Quarterly* 21(2) (1994): 171–86.

Wang, Carolyn C., and Mary Ann Burris. 'Photovoice: Concept, Methodology, and Use for Participatory Needs Assessment.' *Health, Education and Behavior* 24(3) (1997): 369–387.

Wang, Carolyn C., Jennifer L. Cash, and Lisa S. Powers. 'Who Knows the Streets as Well as the Homeless? Promoting Personal and Community Action through Photovoice.' *Health Promotion Practice* 1(1) (2000): 81–9.

Wang, Carolyn C., and Cheri A. Pies. 'Family, Maternal, and Child Health through Photovoice.' *Maternal and Child Care* 8(2) (2004): 95–102.

Wang, Carolyn C., W.K. Yi, Z.W. Tao, and K. Carovano. 'Photovoice as a Participatory Health Promotion Strategy.' *Health Promotion International* 13(1) (1998): 775–86.

Yanos, Philip T., S.M. Barrow, and Sam Tsemberis. 'Community Integration in the Early Phase of Housing among Homeless Persons Diagnosed with Severe Mental Illness: Successes and Challenges.' *Community Mental Health Journal* 40 (2004): 133–50.

Zarb, Gerry. 'On the Road to Damascus: First Steps toward Changing the Relations of Disability Research Production.' *Disability and Society* 7 (1992): 125–38.

Index

Ability Society, 6
addiction. *See* drug and alcohol use
Alberta Mental Health Board
  (AMHB), 70, 74, 103, 132
alcohol. *See* drug and alcohol use
Alexander, Bryant K., 142n7
Ali, Jamal, 5–6, 11, 47, 78, 80, 88, 103,
  106, 111, 112, 113, 115, 119; article in
  the *Calgary Herald*, 4, 6, 114, 131–3;
  article in *Schizophrenia Digest*, 4, 6,
  114–15
Allen, Tom, 150n2
Andreason, Nancy, 145n29
Arney, Laurie, 5, 6, 27, 42, 78, 80, 88,
  93, 94, 99, 107–8, 109, 110, 111, 112,
  113, 114, 115, 119, 149n6; journal
  entries, 37, 38–9, 39–40, 43, 44–5,
  45–6, 47, 48, 83, 84, 85–6, 99–102,
  103–4, 105–6
Assured Income for the Severely
  Handicapped (AISH), 48–9, 67,
  69–71, 72, 77, 90, 105, 126, 127
'author evacuated' text, 95
autoethnography, 142n7

Baker, Tamara A., 151
Balcazar, Fabricio, et al., 142n5

Becker, Harold S., et al., 153n3, 153n6
Benson, George, 5, 6, 38, 50, 106, 111,
  114; journal entry, 44
Beresford, Peter, 117, 142n5, 143n8,
  149n1, 149n2, 154n1
Berger, Lauren, 153n12
Bochner, Arthur P., and Carolyn E.
  Ellis, 142n7, 152n2, 153n6, 153n8
Boote, Jonathan, et al., 149n2
Booth, Tim, and Wendy Booth, 151n6
Bridge to Discharge Project, 14
'broken brain,' 17, 145n29
Burns, Tom, D., et al., 147n51

Calderbank, Cindy, 5, 6, 45, 80, 108,
  110, 113, 114, 115, 116; journal entry,
  44; letter in *Schizophrenia Digest*, 6,
  115
Calgary Association of Self Help, 6
Calgary Herald (articles in), 4, 6, 99,
  114, 129–33, 141n1
California Network of Mental Health
  Clients, 14
Campbell, Jean, and R. Schreiber,
  143n9
Canadian Centre on Disability Studies, 9, 12